NATIONAL ACADEMIES *Sciences Engineering Medicine*

NATIONAL ACADEMIES PRESS
Washington, DC

The Role of Advanced Computation, Predictive Technologies, and Big Data Analytics in Food and Nutrition Research

Alice Vorosmarti and Joe Alper,
Rapporteurs

Food and Nutrition Board

Health and Medicine Division

Proceedings of a Workshop

NATIONAL ACADEMIES PRESS 500 Fifth Street, NW Washington, DC 20001

This activity was supported by contracts between the National Academy of Sciences and Texas A&M Institute for Advancing Health Through Agriculture (AB0767199) and the U.S. Department of Agriculture, Agricultural Research Service (59-0204-0-003). Any opinions, findings, conclusions, or recommendations expressed in this publication do not necessarily reflect the views of any organization or agency that provided support for the project.

International Standard Book Number-13: 978-0-309-71570-6
International Standard Book Number-10: 0-309-71570-9
Digital Object Identifier: https://doi.org/10.17226/27478

This publication is available from the National Academies Press, 500 Fifth Street, NW, Keck 360, Washington, DC 20001; (800) 624-6242 or (202) 334-3313; http://www.nap.edu.

Copyright 2024 by the National Academy of Sciences. National Academies of Sciences, Engineering, and Medicine and National Academies Press and the graphical logos for each are all trademarks of the National Academy of Sciences. All rights reserved.

Printed in the United States of America.

Suggested citation: National Academies of Sciences, Engineering, and Medicine. 2024. *The role of advanced computation, predictive technologies, and big data analytics in food and nutrition research: Proceedings of a workshop.* Washington, DC: The National Academies Press. https://doi.org/10.17226/27478.

The **National Academy of Sciences** was established in 1863 by an Act of Congress, signed by President Lincoln, as a private, nongovernmental institution to advise the nation on issues related to science and technology. Members are elected by their peers for outstanding contributions to research. Marcia McNutt is president.

The **National Academy of Engineering** was established in 1964 under the charter of the National Academy of Sciences to bring the practices of engineering to advising the nation. Members are elected by their peers for extraordinary contributions to engineering. John L. Anderson is president.

The **National Academy of Medicine** (formerly the Institute of Medicine) was established in 1970 under the charter of the National Academy of Sciences to advise the nation on medical and health issues. Members are elected by their peers for distinguished contributions to medicine and health. Victor J. Dzau is president.

The three Academies work together as the **National Academies of Sciences, Engineering, and Medicine** to provide independent, objective analysis and advice to the nation and conduct other activities to solve complex problems and inform public policy decisions. The National Academies also encourage education and research, recognize outstanding contributions to knowledge, and increase public understanding in matters of science, engineering, and medicine.

Learn more about the National Academies of Sciences, Engineering, and Medicine at **www.nationalacademies.org**.

Consensus Study Reports published by the National Academies of Sciences, Engineering, and Medicine document the evidence-based consensus on the study's statement of task by an authoring committee of experts. Reports typically include findings, conclusions, and recommendations based on information gathered by the committee and the committee's deliberations. Each report has been subjected to a rigorous and independent peer-review process and it represents the position of the National Academies on the statement of task.

Proceedings published by the National Academies of Sciences, Engineering, and Medicine chronicle the presentations and discussions at a workshop, symposium, or other event convened by the National Academies. The statements and opinions contained in proceedings are those of the participants and are not endorsed by other participants, the planning committee, or the National Academies.

Rapid Expert Consultations published by the National Academies of Sciences, Engineering, and Medicine are authored by subject-matter experts on narrowly focused topics that can be supported by a body of evidence. The discussions contained in rapid expert consultations are considered those of the authors and do not contain policy recommendations. Rapid expert consultations are reviewed by the institution before release.

For information about other products and activities of the National Academies, please visit www.nationalacademies.org/about/whatwedo.

PLANNING COMMITTEE FOR A WORKSHOP ON THE ROLE OF ADVANCED COMPUTATION, PREDICTIVE TECHNOLOGIES, AND BIG DATA ANALYTICS IN FOOD AND NUTRITION RESEARCH[1]

RODOLPHE BARRANGOU (*Cochair*), Todd R. Klaenhammer Distinguished Professor, North Carolina State University
SHARON I. KIRKPATRICK (*Cochair*), Associate Professor, University of Waterloo
BECCA B. R. JABLONSKI, Codirector, Food Systems Institute, and Associate Professor, Colorado State University
ANANT MADABHUSHI, Robert W. Woodruff Professor and Research Career Scientist, Georgia Institute of Technology and Emory University
CARMEN D. TEKWE, Associate Professor of Biostatistics, Indiana University at Bloomington
DIANA M. THOMAS, Professor, U.S. Military Academy at West Point

Staff

ALICE VOROSMARTI, Associate Program Officer
MELANIE ARTHUR, Senior Program Assistant
ANN L. YAKTINE, Director, Food and Nutrition Board

Consultant

JOE ALPER, writer

---

[1]The National Academies of Sciences, Engineering, and Medicine's planning committees are solely responsible for organizing the workshop, identifying topics, and choosing speakers. The responsibility for the published Proceedings of a Workshop rests with the workshop rapporteurs and the institution.

Reviewers

This Proceedings of a Workshop was reviewed in draft form by individuals chosen for their diverse perspectives and technical expertise. The purpose of this independent review is to provide candid and critical comments that will assist the National Academies of Sciences, Engineering, and Medicine in making each published proceedings as sound as possible and to ensure that it meets the institutional standards for quality, objectivity, evidence, and responsiveness to the charge. The review comments and draft manuscript remain confidential to protect the integrity of the process.

We thank the following individuals for their review of this proceedings:

HOLLY NICASTRO, National Institutes of Health
CHIRAG PATEL, Harvard Medical School
JILL REEDY, National Cancer Institute

Although the reviewers listed above provided many constructive comments and suggestions, they were not asked to endorse the content of the proceedings nor did they see the final draft before its release. The review of this proceedings was overseen by **CATHIE WOTEKI,** Iowa State University. She was responsible for making certain that an independent examination of this proceedings was carried out in accordance with standards of the National Academies and that all review comments were carefully considered. Responsibility for the final content rests entirely with the rapporteurs and the National Academies.

Contents

ACRONYMS AND ABBREVIATIONS   xiii

1   INTRODUCTION   1
Introductory Remarks, 2
Organization of the Proceedings, 8

2   SETTING THE STAGE   9
Highlights from the Presentations of Individual Speakers, 9
AI and Health, 10
Ethics, Privacy, Bias, and Trust in the Application of AI, 14
The Promises and Challenges of AI in Nutrition and Food
    Sciences, 17
Moderated Discussion, 18

3   APPLICATIONS AND LESSONS LEARED   21
Highlights from the Presentations of Individual Speakers, 21
Wearables: Sensors, Images, and AI for Food Intake
    Monitoring, 23
Microbiome and Diet, 26
Quantitative Analysis of Metabolomics Data to Inform
    Precision Health, 30
Applications of AI in Nutrition Research, 34
Designing Nutrition Studies for AI Data Analysis, 39
AI and the Big Challenges in Agriculture and Food, 43

Nourish or Perish: A Research Journey through Food Supply Chains, 47
Reaction to the Presentations on Applications and Lessons Learned, 51
Moderated Discussion, 52

4   CAPACITY BUILDING   57
Highlights from the Presentations of Individual Speakers, 57
Training Program in AI and Precision Nutrition, 58
Building Inclusive Teams for Food and Nutrition Research, 61
Moderated Discussion, 69

5   POTENTIAL APPLICATIONS OF AI TO LARGE-SCALE FOOD AND NUTRITION INITIATIVES   73
Highlights from the Presentations of Individual Speakers, 73
Advancing AI and ML in Biomedical Research and Health Care at NIH, 74
The NIH NPH Program, 77
Ethics, Access, Legal Frameworks, and Fairness in AI, 79
Moderated Discussion, 84

6   FINAL DISCUSSION AND SYNTHESIS   85

REFERENCES   89

APPENDIXES
A   Workshop Agenda   99
B   Biographical Sketches of Speakers and Moderators   105

Box and Figures

BOX

1-1 Workshop Statement of Task, 2

FIGURES

2-1 A fairness tree, 15

3-1 Examples of wearable sensors, 24
3-2 Distribution of known and unknown bioactive molecules in rosemary, 28
3-3 Analytic methods to characterize dietary patterns, 36
3-4 A food network to understand meal patterns, 37
3-5 Natural language processing of tweets reveals geographic differences in food consumption patterns, 38
3-6 Solving the challenges of using AI to enable precision nutrition requires a multiscale, multisystem approach, 40
3-7 The layers that would make up a geographic information system of a human being, 44
3-8 The environmental impacts of food and agriculture, 45
3-9 The widespread effects of food malnutrition, 47
3-10 Negative feedback loops make fruits and vegetables expensive to eat and hard to purchase for low-income populations, 49
3-11 The current food supply chain is primarily inventory pushed and depends on a large number of intermediaries, 49

4-1 Factors associated with the variability between individuals in response to diet, 59
4-2 The overlap of DEI and belonging, 62
4-3 Prevalence of food insecurity by selected household characteristics, 2021, 63
4-4 Bringing the perspective of African American researchers to the problem of excess obesity in African American populations, 64
4-5 Move toward inclusive excellence by promoting and supporting women in science, 68

5-1 The complex nature of farm decisions, 80

Acronyms and Abbreviations

AI	artificial intelligence
AIFS	AI Institute for Next-Generation Food Systems
ARS	Agricultural Research Service
AUC	area under the curve
CDS	clinical decision support
DEI	diversity, equity, and inclusion
DL	deep learning
EHR	electronic health record
FDA	U.S. Food and Drug Administration
IHA	Institute for Advancing Health through Agriculture
LGBTQ+	lesbian, gay, bisexual, transgender, queer/questioning. The + symbol acknowledges that there may be sexual/gender identities not represented in the other terms
ML	machine learning
NCI	National Cancer Institute
NIH	National Institutes of Health
NPH	Nutrition for Precision Health

NUTRISS	Research Center on Nutrition, Health, and Society
ODS	Office of Dietary Supplements
ODSS	Office of Data Science Strategy
PA	placental abruption
PI	principal investigator
RFA	request for applications
STEM	science, technology, engineering, and mathematics
USDA	U.S. Department of Agriculture

1

Introduction[1]

Artificial intelligence (AI), machine learning (ML), and deep learning (DL) have shown promise toward aiding in developing algorithms to better understand and predict interactions between food- and nutrition-related data and health outcomes, particularly when large amounts of data need to be structured and integrated. However, additional research is needed to identify areas where AI/ML are likely to have an impact and their limitations. In addition, federal agencies are interested in exploring criteria around how to best use AI/ML in nutrition research.

To explore current knowledge and practice related to the application of advanced computation, big data analytics, and high-performance computing to support scientific advances in food and nutrition research, the National Academies of Sciences, Engineering, and Medicine's (the National Academies') Food and Nutrition Board convened experts to discuss this and related subjects in Washington, DC, on October 10–11, 2023. The speakers and participants discussed definitions and methods; the appropriate use of evidence generated from these methods to inform food- and nutrition-related programs and policies; considered issues related to diversity, equity, inclusion, bias, and privacy; identified opportunities and challenges related to capacity building and training; and explored the future potential of these

---

[1] The planning committee's role was limited to planning the workshop, and the Proceedings of a Workshop was prepared by the workshop rapporteurs as a factual summary of what occurred at the workshop. Statements, recommendations, and opinions expressed are those of individual presenters and participants and are not necessarily endorsed or verified by the National Academies of Sciences, Engineering, and Medicine, and they should not be construed as reflecting any group consensus.

methods in food and nutrition research. The workshop sessions highlighted applications and lessons learned from studies of AI, ML, and DL methods in both food and nutrition research and other fields. Box 1-1 provides the statement of task for the workshop.

INTRODUCTORY REMARKS

Rodolphe Barrangou, the Todd R. Klaenhammer Distinguished Professor at North Carolina State University and workshop planning committee cochair, welcomed participants and said that the workshop would focus on the future of food and nutrition research and the role that advanced computation, predictive technologies, and big data analytics will play. "We have to talk about challenges and opportunities. We have to talk about building the systems we need to implement that technology," said Barrangou.

Sharon Kirkpatrick, associate professor in the School of Public Health Sciences at the University of Waterloo and workshop planning committee

---

BOX 1-1
Workshop Statement of Task

A planning committee of the National Academies of Sciences, Engineering, and Medicine will plan a 2-day public workshop to explore current knowledge and practice related to the application of advanced computation, big data analytics, and high-performance computing to support scientific advances in food and nutrition research. The workshop will feature invited presentations and discussions that will focus on providing guidance to researchers and policy makers. Topic areas to be considered include

- Definitions and methodology
  - Clear definitions of artificial intelligence (AI) and related activities such as machine learning (ML), deep learning (DL), etc.
  - Common methods, standards, and protocols
  - Role of AI as a tool for developing study design
- Current applications of AI/ML in food and nutrition research
  - Biomarker or bioactive discovery
  - Data collection related to food intake assessment and monitoring methods—tools such as sensors, wearables, smartphone applications
  - Identifying relationship between foods/nutrients and health outcomes
  - Behavioral research—advancing behavior change by teaching personalized health behaviors from personalized data
  - Nutritional quality
  - Food systems
  - Food safety

cochair, summarized what was ahead. The workshop would start by laying a solid foundation in terms of key concepts related to data science; introduce the theme of ethics, privacy, bias, and trust to be considered; explore how data science and AI/ML are being used in nutrition and food sciences; and outline some of the related promises and challenges. The first day would include a session on applications and lessons learned from work on wearables, the microbiome, and metabolomics. The day would end with a session on capacity building and inclusivity. Day 2 would include a second session on applications and lessons learned, focusing on designing nutrition studies for AI data analysis, how to gain farmers' trust in AI, and the application of AI to supply chains. The following session would focus on the potential applications of AI and data science to large-scale initiatives. The final session would feature a broad discussion of the workshop's key themes.

- o Ways that AI is being applied in other disciplines relevant to food and nutrition
- Considerations for diversity, equity, and inclusion
  - o Impact of AI, ML, and DL on underrepresented populations
  - o Bias in development of datasets, algorithms, and applications
  - o Data privacy
- Questions and considerations going forward/research gaps
  - o What is the greatest limitation to AI now in research and what is the future potential?
  - o What is the appropriate use of AI now and in the future? Hypothesis generation? "Evidence" for decision making? Where does it fit on the evidence hierarchy? Classifying subgroups (responders/nonresponders)?
  - o How can AI be used to increase efficiency (costs) and resiliency in the food system?
  - o What is needed to build trust in using advanced computation approaches within the food and nutrition research community?
  - o Workforce needs:
    1. Identify experience and skills for successful research teams. Identify training opportunities/exposure to data science methods for food and nutrition researchers

The planning committee will plan and organize the workshop, select and invite speakers and discussants, and moderate the discussions. A Proceedings-in-Brief for the workshop and a final workshop proceedings of the presentations and discussions will be prepared by a designated rapporteur in accordance with institutional guidelines.

Institute for Advancing Health Through Agriculture

Patrick Stover, director of the Institute for Advancing Health through Agriculture (IHA) at Texas A&M University, said that IHA was created to use systems approaches to reimagine the connections between food and the health of the nation. IHA focuses on precision nutrition, understanding the variability in the diet and disease relationship, responsive agriculture, and healthy living. He defined responsive agriculture as "an agriculture system and food environment that supports health through nutrition for all while ensuring the system is economically robust and environmentally sustainable for future generations" and healthy living as "translating advancements in precision nutrition and responsive agriculture into evidence-based practices and policies to make food and agriculture the solution to skyrocketing health care costs."

This is a critical time for nutrition science and public health nutrition, said Stover. Dietary patterns are a major driver of rising health care costs affecting everyone. Over 70 percent of people in the United States have overweight or obesity, and 60 percent have at least one chronic health condition. "But we also know that we can bring the very best science to bear to achieve solutions to agriculture, food, and nutrition," he said, noting that agriculture has always responded to societal expectations. For example, agriculture and food systems were successfully engineered after World War II to produce calories in abundance, making hunger and food insecurity rare for most households and not the result of insufficient food production. In subsequent decades, research led to understanding nutritional deficiency disorders—"hidden hunger"—and developing population-based guidance and policies that largely prevented them.

The nation faces the challenge of addressing diet-related chronic diseases and has new expectations for food, agriculture, and nutrition. "Including health and chronic disease reduction as goals of food and agriculture will require transformational advances across the entire food and agriculture value chain," said Stover. "The science and policies we use to address hunger and nutritional deficiency disorders are comparatively simple; the diet-related chronic disease connection includes multiple interacting health behaviors and environmental exposures."

At the individual level, one size does not fit all regarding diet–disease or diet–health relationships, adding to the complexity of the challenge. Thus, the same approaches used to address nutritional deficiencies are inadequate to address the variability and dynamics that define the connection between agriculture, food, nutrition, and health. "Making food and agriculture the solution for chronic disease reduction will require new approaches, new types of data, and better ways of communicating dietary information of the public," said Stover. "The expectations are high, and the rigorous science we are going to address today must lead the way." It is critical, he added, to avoid overpromising and get this right to maintain public support.

Stover said that although data science is transforming society and offering solutions to address complexity, the field of food and nutrition is a late adopter. However, advances in AI, including layering numerous associations on validated, physiological, metabolic, or social computational networks, offer the possibility of establishing true causal relationships that underpin connections among agriculture, food, and health.

U.S. Department of Agriculture (USDA) Agricultural Research Service (ARS) Human Nutrition Program

Cindy Davis, national program leader for the USDA-ARS Human Nutrition Program, said that the workshop's topic is exceedingly relevant to her program, whose mission is to define the role of food and its components in optimizing health throughout the life cycle for all Americans by conducting high-national-priority research. AI/ML, she said, has shown promise for developing algorithms to better understand and predict interactions between food- and nutrition-related data and health outcomes, particularly when large amounts of data need to be structured and integrated. However, additional research is needed to identify areas where AI/ML is likely to have an impact and understand their limitations.

ARS, said Davis, is USDA's chief in-house scientific agency focused on finding solutions to agricultural problems and conducting research on individual barriers to consuming a healthy diet and achieving a healthy body weight. Its six human nutrition research centers have a core capability for long-term, multidisciplinary, translational research in high-priority areas to improve the nation's health. Its five priorities for 2024–2029 are

1. Bridging the gap between food production and human health by identifying the agricultural practices influencing the nutritional quality and composition of food and conducting multidisciplinary research to understand the complex interactions within the food system and their effects on human health.
2. Monitoring food composition and the nation's nutrient intake to provide food composition data, determine national food consumption and dietary patterns, and develop improved methods to analyze food and determine food and nutrient intake.
3. Developing the scientific basis for dietary guidance by improving the scientific basis for updating national dietary standards and guidelines, identifying mechanisms whereby food, food components, and physical activity promote health, and using advanced

technology to develop and integrate multiple data sources to more precisely inform nutritional requirements.
4. Preventing diet-related chronic disease by identifying mechanisms by which food, food components, and physical activity can help and developing and evaluating diet and physical activity strategies.
5. Understanding life-stage nutrition and metabolism.

Davis noted an increasing recognition that understanding the connections and synergies between nutritional health and agriculture can be achieved only through the broad framework of food systems and simultaneous research across all pillars of the food system. Consensus is emerging that food systems contain four primary, interactive, and interdependent components: human nutrition/health, food production and agriculture, food technology's effects on the environment and vice versa, and consumer choices and attitudes. Understanding the complex interactions within the food system related to human health requires multidisciplinary teams that assess inputs and effects from all sectors. Davis stated that advanced computation, predictive technologies, and big data analytics, of which AI and ML are examples, are necessary to integrate these data.

The U.S. food supply, said Davis, is fluid, and providing timely and accurate food composition data is complex because of constant changes in food regulations and policy, food choices and consumer preferences, production and processing methods that induce compositional variability, and demographic changes in the population. In addition, food composition and food intake data are only as accurate as the methods used to obtain them, making advances in instrumentation, analytical procedures, and methodology necessary to provide high-quality data.

Davis noted that the field's understanding of the food-related physiologic processes underlying health and the prevention of disease is expanding constantly. "We are faced with the need to accumulate new information relating to how dietary patterns, specific foods, nutrients, bioactive components, and physical activity influence these processes," she said. In addition, emerging evidence suggests that many subpopulations have differential responses to diet and chronic disease risk and that the large interindividual variability and individual responses to diets and environment are not well characterized.

The increase in diet-related chronic diseases is complex and has multiple etiologies, said Davis. The field appreciates that individual, genetic, epigenetic, phenotypic, social, and microbiome differences influence how dietary intake and physical activity affect health. "Decades of human nutrition research and advances in information technology have left us with substantial amounts of data potentially relevant to human nutritional requirements, but assimilating and using these data has been problematic," said Davis. Recent advances in information technology, including AI/ML, now offer possibilities of searching massive and disparate datasets and integrating multidimensional data on diet, genetics, epigenetics, microbiome, environmental factors, and other factors into a coherent framework.

Science Informing Policy

Jennifer Tiller, deputy staff director for the House Committee on Agriculture, said that her work operationalizing workforce development programs showed her that sometimes policy makers and agencies with the best intentions do not always get policies right because they were not supported by data. While considering reauthorization of the Farm Bill, Congress will deliberate, debate, and draft policies that will affect every part of the agricultural value chain. The House committee chair, she said, firmly believes that policy should use the best science—not political science—and has called for improved nutrition policies that can mitigate increasing instances of diet-related chronic disease among the population served by the programs the committee authorizes.

Tiller said that the largest of these is the Supplemental Nutrition Assistance Program, which serves over 41 million people at an annual cost of $115 billion. Previous testimony before the committee explained that the right resources, research, data, modernized programming, technology, and appropriate and effective federal dietary policy will enable USDA, the states, communities, and academia to improve the nutrition of the millions of Americans who rely on this program. "Every corner of the value chain needs to ensure there is a range of tools to help individuals from all walks of life prevent and conquer instances of disease," said Tiller.

She noted that obesity costs the nation approximately $147 billion in annual health care costs. It also affects quality of life, general longevity, and everything from employment to military readiness. "What we consume matters, and strong, scientifically rigorous federal dietary policy is important to course correct," she said, "No more are programs under the [House] committee's jurisdiction only about hunger. They are now about health, and I think everyone in this room welcomes that evolution."

Something equally important to what Americans consume is educating those who consume, said Tiller. Millions of low-income families participate in a range of nutrition education programming every year. Each program has different rubrics to capture data and measure outcomes, resulting in a questionable effect on those who need this information and education the most. "There exists a critical need for common metrics and an evaluation framework that allows the agencies with oversight of these important programs to house a repository of data that can change our programming for the better," said Tiller. AI/ML have the potential to streamline and synthesize scientific advances that can increase the credibility and transparency of dietary guidance to improve the health of our nation.

ORGANIZATION OF THE PROCEEDINGS

This Proceedings of a Workshop summarizes the presentations. The speakers, panelists, and participants presented a broad range of views and ideas. Following this introductory chapter, Chapter 2 summarizes three presentations that set the stage for the workshop. Chapter 3 recounts the discussions about applications of advanced computation, big data analytics, and high-performance computing and lessons learned. Chapters 4 and 5 report on the discussions about capacity building and potential AI applications to large-scale food and nutrition initiatives, respectively. The final chapter presents a synthesis of the workshop's key ideas to move the field forward. Appendixes A and B contain the agenda and biographical sketches of the speakers and session moderators, respectively. The speakers' presentations (as PDF and video files) have been archived.[2]

---

[2] Available at https://www.nationalacademies.org/event/40460_10-2023_the-role-of-advanced-computation-predictive-technologies-and-big-data-analytics-related-to-food-and-nutrition-research-a-workshop (accessed January 9, 2024).

2

Setting the Stage

> **Highlights from the Presentations of Individual Speakers**[a]
> - Unsupervised, black-box algorithms lack interpretability of the representations that neural networks generate from data, which can result in a catastrophic failure. (Madabhushi)
> - AI is not magic, and it needs to be used thoughtfully and intentionally when developing algorithms. Interpretability, reproducibility, and equity are key considerations. (Madabhushi)
> - Although DL/AI algorithms can provide a great deal of information about patients, they can perpetuate bias and disparities when deployed widely. (Gichoya)
> - Serious questions arise regarding privacy and regulation of AI systems, such as how and when to get consent for data sharing, are institutional review boards empowered to protect patient privacy in the era of AI, is it possible to sufficiently deidentify and anonymize patients, can patients opt out of data sharing, and is it different to get consent for data from an electronic health record (EHR) versus patient images. (Gichoya)
> - Application of AI in nutrition research has a great potential to increase the capacity to manage and analyze big datasets and perhaps identify new relationships and patterns in diet, but it is difficult because of the complexities and difficulties in measur-

ing relevant characteristics and relating them to the behaviors and societal factors that influence how and what people eat. (Lamarche)
- It is important to develop a common language and culture for the many disciplines that will use AI/ML in food and nutrition research. (Lamarche, Madabhushi)

[a] This list is the rapporteurs' summary of points made by the individual speakers identified, and the statements have not been endorsed or verified by the National Academies of Sciences, Engineering, and Medicine. They are not intended to reflect a consensus among workshop participants.

AI AND HEALTH

Anant Madabhushi, the Robert W. Woodruff Professor and research neuroscientist in the Departments of Biomedical Engineering, Radiology, and Imaging Sciences and Biomedical Informatics and Pathology at both Georgia Tech and Emory University, said that artificial intelligence (AI) has implications for a wide range of areas, including health care, education, and agriculture. His research group has been examining the use of AI with computational imaging technologies for developing better diagnostic, prognostic, and predictive tools capable of identifying the presence or absence of disease and predicting disease outcome, progression, and response to treatment and other interventions. He noted that "precision medicine" refers to the development of prognostic and predictive tools for tailoring therapy for a patient based on their specific risk profile.

Madabhushi explained that deep learning (DL) serves as the foundational architecture of large language models, such as ChatGPT, and refers to a particular variety of machine learning (ML) algorithms. DL algorithms are based on neural networks. Although researchers have been working on neural networks for over 60 years, it has only been with the advent of more powerful computers that they have been able to stack them in sophisticated and complex ways, with individual neurons in the network coding for representations of the data. "You now have the ability to absorb and ingest large amounts of data and learn from those large amounts of data to be able to create these networks that are then able to make predictions based off the data that is being ingested," said Madabhushi.

As an example of how his team has applied this approach to medicine, Madabhushi cited using DL to detect malignant cells in breast pathology images (Lu et al., 2016; Xu et al., 2016; Zhang et al., 2016). With annotations of individual cells in an image of a scanned pathology slide, the network can learn which representations best distinguish a cell of interest from all other cells. Those patterns, he said, are encoded within the individual neurons in the neural network. Each encoded representation is generated automatically by the algorithms that make up the DL framework. "There is no explicit knowledge or explicit predicate features that are being provided to the neural network," said Madabhushi. "The neural network is learning this in an unsupervised manner." The network learned the representations that best describe individual cells and then predicted the precise location of these cells on new images.

The advantage of this type of algorithm, Madabhushi explained, is that it is data driven. In other words, without having any knowledge of breast cancer or pathology, Madabhushi's students were able to create the algorithm and identify individual cells. The caveat is that the representations the network is learning from the data are abstract, and because it generates representations that lack interpretability, these algorithms are often called "mysterious machines" or "black boxes." This lack of interpretability can result in a catastrophic failure.

For example, Madabhushi's team attempted to build a DL neural network to predict the presence of heart failure from endomyocardial biopsies (Nirschl et al., 2018). His collaborators at the University of Pennsylvania provided digital images of pathology slides of endomyocardial biopsies from 100 patients and noted whether heart failure was present. His team used the annotated images to train a neural network, and the resulting weakly supervised algorithms, so called because they develop without detailed information, had free rein to learn features on each pathology slide.

With the algorithm training complete, his collaborators sent slides from a different set of 100 patients. As a check, two cardiac pathologists reviewed the same slides and made their own predictions. The DL network's predictions were 97 percent accurate, and the expert pathologists were only 74 percent accurate. However, when his collaborators sent another set of images, the algorithm's accuracy fell to 75 percent, raising the question of why the performance had dropped so precipitously. The slide scanner had received a software upgrade, which subtly changed the appearance of the individual slides. From a human perspective, the change was unnoticeable, but for the ML network, it was sufficient to diminish performance significantly. "This goes back to this issue of interpretability, because if you do not really understand fundamentally what the network is picking up, then you can have examples of these catastrophic failures where the network suddenly fails," he explained.

Madabhushi cited another research group's work developing a DL algorithm to distinguish between a wolf and a husky (Ribeiro et al., 2016). The investigators trained the algorithm using pictures from the Internet;

when tested against a separate set of images, it was 99 percent accurate, which was surprising because it is hard for humans to tell these two animals apart. However, the network was not picking up any features of the animals' faces but rather whether the picture's background showed snow. "The network had latched onto features that were completely unexpected, and this reiterates the issue of the lack of interpretability, because sometimes it may work but it is not working for the reasons that you would expect," said Madabhushi.

Cynthia Rudin at Duke University has spoken eloquently, said Madabhushi, about the need to exercise care when imbuing interpretability into black-box models, particularly for high-stakes decisions (Rudin, 2019). She called for focusing on inherently interpretable approaches and designing models with intentional interpretable attributes or hallmarks built into them.

Madabhushi listed key considerations for developing AI tools for precision medicine and precision nutrition. The first is interpretability and developing handcrafted, engineered approaches that start with a set of attributes or features with more inherent interpretability. A second consideration is affordability and taking advantage of routinely acquired data, particularly in low- and middle-income countries that may lack the ability to acquire sophisticated data or sophisticated technology to acquire more data. The third consideration is equity and whether an algorithm works across populations or is biased toward a particular population.

One example of his group's work that tries to accommodate these considerations involved leveraging the power of AI to identify lung cancer and the associated tumor habitat using interpretable, noninvasive radiomic biomarkers. Instead of merely providing slide images and letting the algorithm learn unsupervised, Madabhushi's group identified individual cells, different tissue compartments, the architectural arrangement of different cell types, the network arrangements between different cell types, the shape of individual cells, and the appearance of the different tissue compartments in which these cells reside. Using these more interpretable features produced more accurate predictions, enabled determining the tumor phenotype, and segmented out the tumor-associated habitat (Bera et al., 2022).

His team has applied this more intentional approach to a variety of diseases and therapeutic regimens. Using routinely acquired data, such as radiologic scans and pathology images, the resulting algorithms can make predictions of therapeutic response. For example, his team developed an algorithm capable of predicting which women with breast cancer would have short-term versus long-term survival from one specific tumor feature: whether collagen fibers were ordered or disordered (Li, H. et al., 2020, 2021b). Those with disordered collagen had a better prognosis and longer survival, which makes sense given that ordered collagen tends to promote metastasis.

Madabhushi said that the image-based assay also provided significant additional value to more expensive molecular-based tests. Specifically, image classification identified a subset of patients (12 percent of those designated as having a low risk of premature death by the molecular test) who had significantly worse outcomes, suggesting that they should have received chemotherapy. Conversely, the image classifier identified 58 percent of those whom the molecular test identified as high risk and candidates for chemotherapy who actually had significantly lower risk and could possibly have avoided chemotherapy.

It is important, said Madabhushi, to develop more population-tailored models and AI algorithms that account for differences among populations. His team has developed such a model for uterine cancer, which has subtle differences between Black and White patients (Azarianpour Esfahani et al., 2021), that produces more accurate predictions for both Black and White people compared to population-agnostic models. Similarly, an AI-powered model of immune cell architecture extracted from uterine cancers accurately predicted prognostic differences between African and European American patients. They also developed a population-tailored model for breast cancer, which has differences between South Asian and North American patients (Li, H. et al., 2021a).

Another AI-powered algorithm his team developed was able to quantitatively and accurately capture the amount of liver fat from computed tomography scans (Modanwal et al., 2020). "What has been interesting is that we are starting to see a strong association between the AI-quantified liver fat and cardiovascular disease," said Madabhushi. His team has validated this algorithm in some 47,000 patients. By leveraging standard ultrasound images, they also developed an AI-powered algorithm that can predict major adverse cardiovascular events in chronic kidney disease patients (Dhamdhere et al., 2023) and another that uses twistedness of the vessels in the eye to predict response to therapies for eye disease (Dong et al., 2022). Recent data suggest that vessel twistedness might be able to predict Alzheimer's disease and heart disease.

Madabhushi said that AI is not magic. It needs to be used thoughtfully and intentionally when developing algorithms, with interpretability, reproducibility, and equity being key considerations. Unsupervised and supervised AI approaches provide a trade-off between not requiring domain knowledge and interpretability, but independent of the approach, rigorous validation is needed across different test sites. Finally, it is crucial to create carefully curated, representative, and inclusive training datasets for AI and nutrition.

ETHICS, PRIVACY, BIAS, AND TRUST IN THE APPLICATION OF AI

Judy Gichoya, associate professor of interventional radiology and informatics at Emory University, said that applying AI to predictive nutrition will be a bigger, more difficult task compared to using it with imaging data. She noted the harm of not sharing health data and that inequitable data access may lead to expensive and adverse data outcomes.

Gichoya said that it is difficult for experts to agree on what a fair algorithm is and whether it is fair to an individual or a group (see Figure 2-1). She showed examples of unfairness. In one case, where researchers examined the accuracy of four DL models designed to segment cardiac magnetic resonance images, all four models had performance biases depending on whether the images came from a man or woman or a Black versus a White individual (Lee et al., 2023).

In another case, a DL model for analyzing chest radiographs severely underdiagnosed underserved patient populations, including women, Black individuals, and people on Medicaid (Seyyed-Kalantari et al., 2021). Moreover, intersectionality was an issue: a Black woman on Medicaid, for example, had the greatest possibility of being underdiagnosed, but the model produced better results for Black women on private insurance. This intersectionality arises because of the interactions of many factors in an individual's life and how those factors change across the lifespan. "This intersectionality is something we still do not understand regarding how to evaluate for fairness, especially when we are trying to fit this to a single mathematical function," said Gichoya.

She also cited a study showing that a commercial algorithm used to determine who is eligible to be referred to managed care and receive home health care rather than return to the hospital is severely biased by race (Obermeyer et al., 2019). This research showed that Black patients assigned the same level of risk as White patients by the algorithm are actually sicker. The investigators determined that bias happens because the algorithm treats health costs as a proxy for health needs. Less money is spent on Black patients with the same level of need, so the algorithm falsely concludes that they are healthier than White patients who are equally sick.

She mentioned another example in which AI biased the human experts. In this work, investigators presented radiologists with a set of mammograms along with a correct assessment provided by an AI system and another set accompanied by an incorrect AI-generated assessment (Dratsch et al., 2023). With bad information, the radiologists' performance fell. In other words, AI-generated information biased the radiologists, leading them to discount their own expertise. "What is surprising is [that] you can mislead the most experienced people based on the type of output and when you integrate AI," said Gichoya.

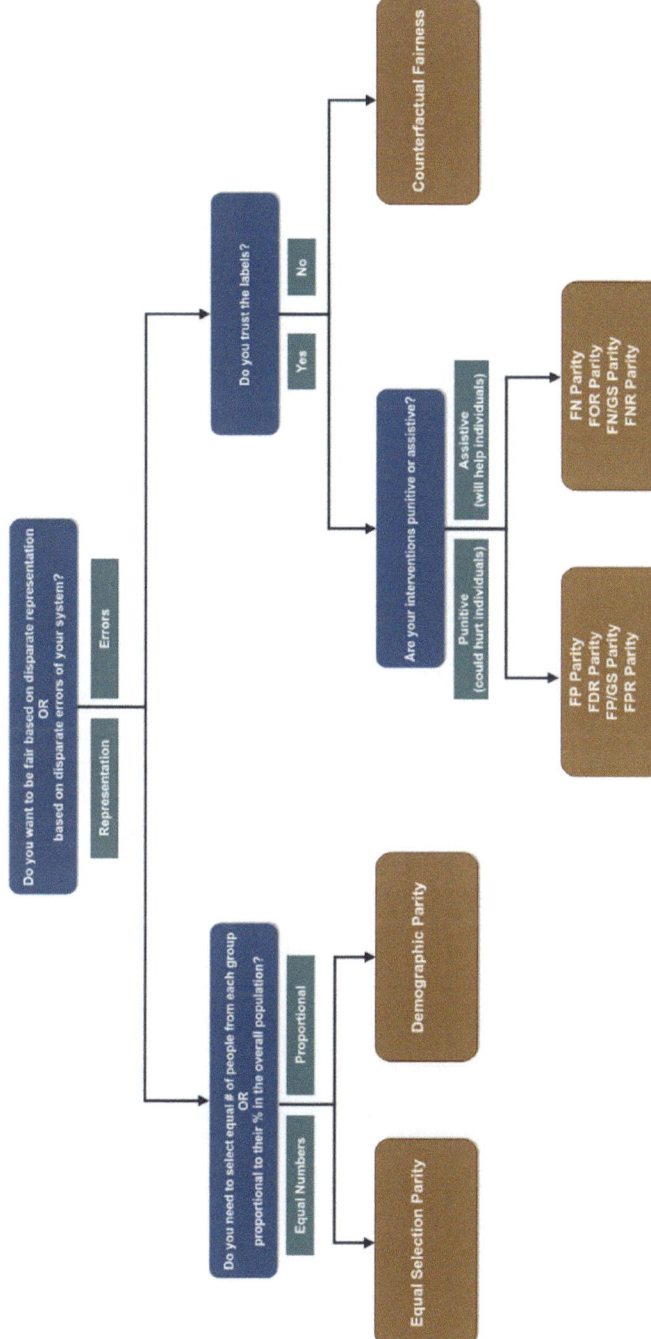

FIGURE 2-1 A fairness tree.
SOURCE: Presented by Judy Gichoya on October 10, 2024, at the workshop on The Role of Advanced Computation, Predictive Technologies, and Big Data Analytics in Food and Nutrition Research; Saleiro et al., 2018.

Turning to the subject of bias in data collection, Gichoya said that investigators can introduce bias in their data depending on how they assemble a dataset. For example, in imaging studies, the investigators might not image all eligible patients or could inadvertently include mislabeled images that skew the dataset (Drukker et al., 2023). Using an incomplete set of possible labels when characterizing the information-dense images that inform ML models leads to a phenomenon known as "hidden stratification" (Oakden-Rayner et al., 2020).

As an example, she described a study in which researchers developed AI systems that appeared to accurately detect COVID-19 in chest X-rays. However, closer examination found that these systems were relying on confounding factors rather than actual pathology, similar to the results Madabhushi noted in his wolf–husky example. As a result, said Gichoya, these systems failed when tested with images from a different hospital (DeGrave et al., 2021).

Gichoya cited a study by herself and her collaborators in which they detected racial and ethnic health disparities using DL with chest X-rays and compared the results to administrative diagnostic codes in COVID-19 patients (Pyrros et al., 2022). The discrepancy between the model's assessment and the administrative code was associated with language preference or a social deprivation index, suggesting that it is an independent predictor of health disparities.

In other studies, she and her collaborators were able to detect type 2 diabetes using DL informed by frontal chest X-rays (Pyrros et al., 2023) and identify a patient's race (Gichoya et al., 2022). Similarly, other groups have shown that DL models could predict health care expenses (Sohn et al., 2022) and estimate biological age (Mitsuyama et al., 2023; Raghu et al., 2021) from chest X-rays. One of the latter studies also found that the DL-based chest X-ray age could predict long-term all-cause and cardiovascular mortality (Raghu et al., 2021). She noted the difficulty of explaining these results and emphasized that although these algorithms can provide a great deal of information, they can perpetuate bias and disparities when deployed widely.

Gichoya concluded by acknowledging that the federal government is focusing on discrimination and bias in AI systems. At the same time, serious questions arise regarding their privacy and regulation, such as how and when is consent needed for data sharing, are institutional review boards empowered to protect patient privacy in the era of AI, is it possible to sufficiently deidentify and anonymize patients, can patients opt out of sharing their data, and is there a mechanism to obtain partial consent versus no consent for sensitive patient images.

THE PROMISES AND CHALLENGES OF AI IN NUTRITION AND FOOD SCIENCES

Benoît Lamarche, professor in the School of Nutrition at Université Laval and scientific director and founder of the Nutrition, Health, and Society Center (NUTRISS), said that the center focuses on precision nutrition, eating behaviors, and nutrition and society. He noted that AI has great potential in nutrition research, but it is difficult because of the complexities and difficulties in measuring relevant characteristics and relating them to the behaviors and societal factors that influence how and what people eat.

Lamarche explained that with traditional statistics, researchers take their data, decide that the model will be to explain those data, and then use the model to predict an outcome. With AI/ML/DL methods, the data and results are the inputs, and the output is the model that makes predictions. He noted that AI, as with traditional statistics, follows the garbage in, garbage out paradigm. For example, the Canadian National Health Survey on Nutrition uses 24-hour recall as its data source. Robust ways exist to deal with measurement error and under- or overreporting of food and energy intakes using sophisticated statistical methods. Overlooking these errors with AI-based methods may introduce bias into the final model with unknown consequences for the results. This is problematic because data show, for example, that underreporting is not systematic across all foods people report to have eaten, with a large proportion of it related to specific foods, particularly low-quality foods. Measurement errors make the "image" of dietary intake fuzzy, akin to pictures with poor-quality pixels, for which AI-based methods have limited capacity.

Nevertheless, AI shows promise to enhance nutrition research, such as by increasing the capacity to manage and analyze big datasets and perhaps identify new relationships and patterns in diet (Côté and Lamarche, 2021; Kirk et al., 2022). Combining genetics, dietary intake, and social and demographic data may provide a better understanding of dietary patterns and enable more accurate prediction of health outcomes. It may be that people taking pictures of their meals with a smartphone can provide enough data for AI approaches to identify dietary patterns. However, this would have limitations. For example, a photo showing a plate of spaghetti and meatballs does not reveal how much meat or vegetable protein is in the sauce or how much salt the meal contains. Other challenges include the need to standardize methods, build capacity, and develop a new vocabulary and for nutrition researchers to understand the culture of AI researchers and vice versa. For example, p values and collinearity are generally not problematic in AI-based methods, which researchers used to traditional statistical methods must adapt to (Côté et al., 2022).

Non-image-based methods may also provide useful data to power AI models, said Lamarche. For example, devices attached to eyeglasses can estimate how long a person is chewing foods by detecting facial movements. However, they cannot tell what the person is chewing or how much food they have actually consumed on one occasion or over a longer term.

Lamarche reinforced the need to standardize dietary patterns methods and scores to advance the field (Reedy et al., 2018). There is also a need to develop methods and models that capture the totality of the diet and to evaluate the effect of measurement error and develop methods to adjust for this error.

Capacity building will be key, said Lamarche. In collaboration with the Sorbonne, NUTRISS held a boot camp in 2023 that brought together AI and nutrition researchers. The two sets of experts worked together to learn each other's vocabulary and culture; in hands-on activities, nutrition students learned to code different algorithms and the AI engineers learned what to do with the data the algorithms produced.

MODERATED DISCUSSION

Rodolphe Barrangou, the moderator, asked the panelists to name the biggest opportunity or challenge. Madabhushi replied that the biggest opportunity is the ability to take advantage of routinely acquired data that are not being exploited. The challenge will be identifying and pulling together equitable and representative datasets from multiple institutions. Gichoya called the challenge of using AI in nutrition research a "moonshot problem" because it is so big and complex. "I am not so sure, as an AI researcher, that AI is the solution if we cannot figure out the data and the standards," she said. To Lamarche, the opportunity lies in changing the perspective on the link between diet and health and ensuring that researchers who move into this area are mindful of the limitations of the available data. He also noted the opportunity to learn more about the intricacies of diet and health, although AI will not get people to eat more fruits and vegetables.

Barrangou asked the panel about reconciling the problem of having a wealth of diverse existing datasets yet wanting data to be standardized. "Is it a matter of restructuring data we already have and parsing it out in certain formats, or do we need to rethink how we collect data and start from scratch?" he asked. Gichoya replied that it is impossible to start from scratch and will be difficult to agree on standards, making efforts to harmonize datasets critically important.

Madabhushi agreed that trying to fit standards to existing data will be challenging, but the opportunity is to think intentionally about the standards, qualifications, and guardrails needed for the data to be useful for AI models. Lamarche noted the need to develop a culture for these nutrition studies, which will require a big community of people starting to think in a concerted manner about data limitations and how to deal with them. Both Madabhushi and Lamarche pointed to the need to develop a common language the nutrition and AI communities can use.

Where the AI field can help, said Lamarche, is taking individual data, connecting them with the variables that influence individual choice, and identifying actionable variables or features that public health can use to educate the public and change behavior. Madabhushi commented that the examples he and Gichoya shared produce correlations and not causative associations. Over time, AI may be able to generate causative associations, but meanwhile, correlations may be sufficient to develop intervention trials based on evidence, he said. Historically, Barrangou added, nutrition research has established correlations rather than causation, but AI may develop some ability to predict outcomes that can enable preventive interventions. Madabhushi added that AI-generated risk predictions could inform educational efforts to change behaviors or even help point to healthier alternatives that could replace nutritionally poor foods.

Barrangou asked the panelists for their ideas about how to build the multidisciplinary teams needed to advance the field. One approach Gichoya has used is to hold a datathon, which brings together people from a range of fields—clinicians, data scientists, programmers, AI experts, social scientists, and others—to work on a large set of real-world patient data from a variety of perspectives. This has been a successful model that has started new partnerships and brought new researchers into the field.

3

Applications and Lessons Learned

> **Highlights from the Presentations of Individual Speakers**[a]
> - Wearables allow for "passive" detection of eating events but by themselves may not provide insights of the foods being consumed. (Sazonov)
> - AI and ML methods form the backbone of technology-based dietary and behavioral assessment, but many technical issues have yet to be resolved, and ethical and privacy issues need to be addressed. (Sazonov)
> - The microbiome and diet are intimately linked. (Knight)
> - ML/AI methods are critical for microbiome analysis, and many of the principles likely apply to other multivariate datasets, such as for food. (Knight)
> - Ethical considerations with microbiome interventions, especially around bias, stratification, and safety, also likely apply to dietary intervention. (Knight)
> - Addressing metabolic issues that were once rare but are more prevalent today may be possible through a better understanding of how nutrition affects the microbiome and today's common chronic diseases. (Knight)
> - Exposome research is key to informing precision nutrition by providing an understanding about how exposures and pertur-

bations in endogenous metabolism are linked to an individual's genetics and states of health and wellness. (McRitchie)
- When developing dietary signatures using either untargeted or targeted metabolomics without carefully controlling the diet, the signature may not be accurate. (Lamarche)
- AI has great potential for the nutrition field, but significant challenges must be addressed, such as appropriately considering the quality of the data, developing a common language between nutrition and computational science, and standardizing methods and approaches. (Lamarche)
- Human studies will always have missing data, which can lead to biased and misleading results. (Das)
- Public funding of ethical technologies to benefit society is imperative, particularly when solving problems arising from negative externalities and supercharging positive externalities. (Smith)
- The main barriers to adoption of AI in agriculture are not related to issues of trust but whether AI will solve real-life problems. (Smith)
- A priority should be to invest in problems beset by externalities and develop technologies in those contexts that can help surmount the challenges of human behavior, a much better path than trying to figure out ways to manipulate human behavior. (Smith)
- A lack of data can make it challenging to support historically disadvantaged and underserved farmers and ranchers without exacerbating existing challenges. (Jablonski)
- It is important to show the intended beneficiaries of a model the evidence used to power it and generate ideas that can improve the end user's situation. (Jablonski)
- Develop tutorials written in accessible language that identify limitations of the different methods, how to properly use a method, and how big a sample is necessary. (McRitchie)
- Addressing the scope of AI and ML projects requires a multidisciplinary approach that involves all of the research areas and creates a transdisciplinary approach requiring awareness and the resources to support it. (Das)
- Accessing data from private entities, including farmers and consumers, continues to be a challenge because of issues of ownership and who will profit from the information. (Smith)

- The key to getting entities to share their data is to show them the benefits for them of doing so and create a safe haven for data sharing. (Dugundji)

a This list is the rapporteurs' summary of points made by the individual speakers identified, and the statements have not been endorsed or verified by the National Academies of Sciences, Engineering, and Medicine. They are not intended to reflect a consensus among workshop participants.

WEARABLES: SENSORS, IMAGES, AND AI FOR FOOD INTAKE MONITORING

Edward Sazonov, the James R. Cudworth Endowed Professor in the Department of Electrical and Computer Engineering and head of the Computer Laboratory of Ambient and Wearable Systems at the University of Alabama, said that the first and simplest task to perform with a wearable device (see Figure 3-1) is to detect when and perhaps how much someone is eating. For infants, for example, monitoring sucking or swallowing would be effective (Farooq et al., 2015). Detecting hand gestures or chewing would be easy in a slightly older child.

For older children and adults, hand-to-mouth monitors could provide information about eating (Dong et al., 2012), but they would have relatively low accuracy because of the similarity to everyday gestures and provide no insights into the type of food consumed, said Sazonov. Swallowing monitors worn around an individual's neck would provide a reliable way to detect food and beverage consumption, but people do not like wearing such devices, and they also do not identify food type (Farooq et al., 2014; Kalantarian et al., 2015; Kandori et al., 2012; Makeyev et al., 2012). Chewing monitors are reliable for detecting food and beverage consumption, although sipping beverages may generate false negatives and chewing gum or lip biting may generate false positives, and they would not provide information about food type (Farooq and Sazonov, 2017; Hossain et al., 2023; Päßler et al., 2012; Sazonov and Fontana, 2012).

Sazonov explained that machine learning (ML) and artificial intelligence (AI) models should employ supervised learning given the importance of providing labels for when a person is eating or not and the type of food they are eating. Data collection, cleaning and labeling the data, feature extractions, and model training and validation are critical steps. The limitation of using ML/AI with wearable devices is that only simple, small models can be deployed. Sophisticated and computationally intensive models require the

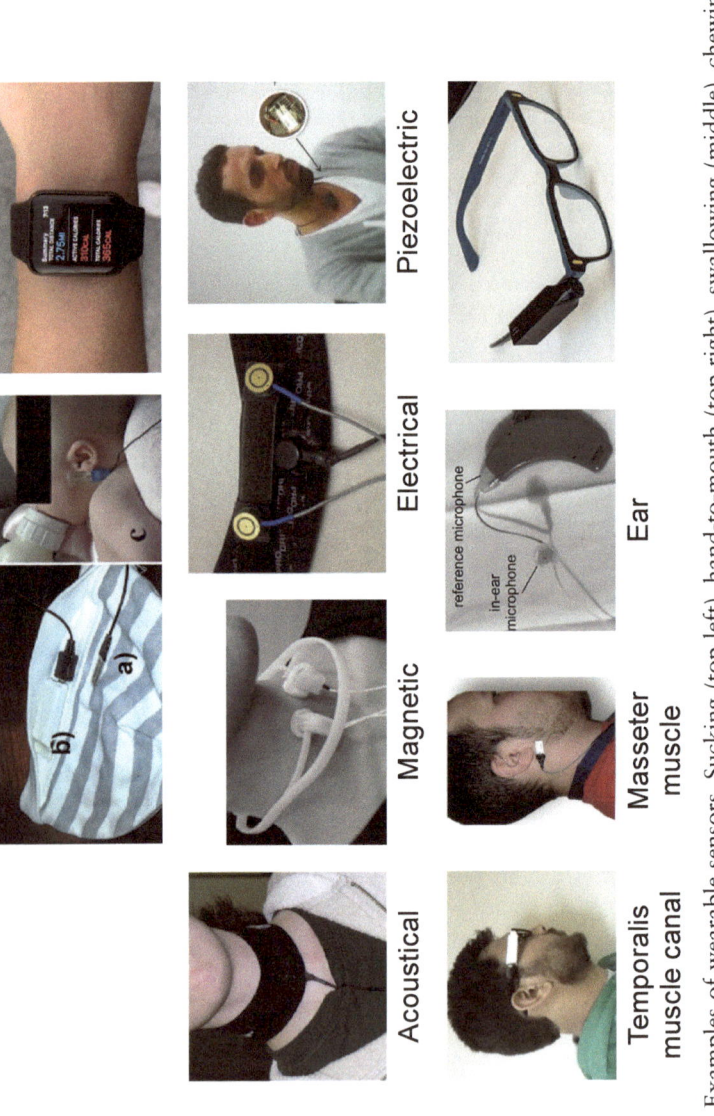

FIGURE 3-1 Examples of wearable sensors. Sucking (top left), hand-to-mouth (top right), swallowing (middle), chewing (bottom left), and image-capturing (bottom right).
SOURCE: Adapted from materials presented by Edward Sazonov on October 10, 2024, at the workshop on The Role of Advanced Computation, Predictive Technologies, and Big Data Analytics in Food and Nutrition Research; Farooq et al., 2014, 2015; Kalantarian et al., 2015; Kandoori et al., 2012; Makeyev et al., 2012.

edge or the cloud, so the device must have network connectivity (Sabry et al., 2022). The beauty of wearable devices is they can provide information via passive detection so participants do not have to report eating events. Wearables can measure the timing and duration of eating, evaluate daily eating patterns, and evaluate the microstructure of eating—the number of bouts, hand gesture rate, chewing rate, and speed, for example (Doulah et al., 2017).

Another capability of wearables, said Sazonov, is estimating the amount of food consumed by connecting the number of hand gestures, bites, chews, and swallows to both the mass and energy content of the food (Dong et al., 2012; Yang et al., 2019). Some wearables, he noted, can take pictures of what the wearer is eating (Liu et al., 2012; Sun et al., 2014). A device his group has developed attaches to an eyeglass temple and captures images of the wearer's food, reveals the eating progression, and automatically detects eating, capturing images of food intake (Doulah et al., 2021). When an ML algorithm running on the device decides that a person is eating, it takes a picture of the food. A nutritionist or image recognition system then analyzes the images to identify the type of food and portion size, although the error rate for both can be large (Doulah et al., 2022; Martin et al., 2009). Sazonov said that an ML algorithm for image-based food classification can be more accurate and provide additional insights (Lo et al., 2020).

Food detection, explained Sazonov, can be achieved by classifying images as food and nonfood, identifying instances of food objects in an image, and identifying the type of food (Chen et al., 2021). A deep learning (DL) algorithm can transform images into text descriptions and provide a synopsis (Qiu et al., 2023). AI can also transform a food image into a recipe that would identify its ingredients (Marin et al., 2021). Sazonov said that segmenting food images is challenging but important for estimating the portion size for each individual food item (He et al., 2013; Wu et al., 2021b), perhaps the most difficult problem for image analysis (Bathgate et al., 2017). A common approach is to have a participant place a fiducial marker in the image for size reference. Images of leftovers provide estimates of the amount consumed. Another approach is to use monocular vision; with the distance from the camera to the food, it can provide an estimate of portion size.

Natural food behavior, said Sazonov, is significantly more complex than commonly used staged food scenes. Food items, for example, can be occluded or consumed in the same bite with other foods. People consume food in many environments and may eat from shared plates. A dimensional reference is not always available, either. Compliance with wearing a device can be a problem, and eating out of protocol is common. It is possible to assess protocol compliance from image and sensor data, he added (Ghosh et al., 2021).

Using images raises privacy concerns, and images may contain information protected by the Health Insurance Portability and Accountability

Act. Sazonov noted that privacy issues are not limited to personal cameras, given the one surveillance camera for every 6.5 people in the United States. Recommendations exist for using wearable cameras in health behavior research (Kelly et al., 2013), as do privacy-preserving techniques for image analysis (Hassan and Sazonov, 2020). Imaging also has inherent limitations, particularly regarding similar-looking items having different nutritional value, such as a gallon of whole versus nonfat milk.

MICROBIOME AND DIET

Rob Knight, the Wolfe Family Endowed Chair of Microbiome Research at Rady's Children's Hospital of San Diego and director of the Center for Microbiome Innovation and professor of pediatrics, bioengineering, data science, and computer science and engineering at the University of California, San Diego (UCSD), said that the dramatic reduction in the cost of DNA sequencing has enabled many of the new applications of microbiome research and generated an enormous amount of data. With all of these data comes the ability to build predictive models for many traits related to health and the microbiome. "Today, I can tell you with about 90 percent accuracy if you are lean or obese solely based on the DNA of the microbes in your gut," said Knight. In comparison, using an individual's DNA sequence to determine whether they are lean or obese is only 57 percent accurate (Knights et al., 2011; Loos, 2012).

Some microbiome patterns, said Knight, are so easy to understand that a human can decipher them without advanced computational techniques. For example, the microbiomes of individuals from Africa, South America, and the United States all converge from the infant to the adult stage within 3 years (Yatsunenko et al., 2012). That raises the question whether the microbiome is set by age 3, which his group addressed by examining microbiome samples from tens of thousands of citizen science participants. The results showed that the microbiome changes with age in adults are so subtle that humans cannot detect a meaningful pattern (de la Cuesta-Zuluaga et al., 2019). However, using the IBM AutoAI system, Knight's group determined a person's age to within 12 years from a stool sample, 5 years from a saliva sample, and 4 years from a skin sample. "Your microbiome provides a detailed readout of your age, just like many other biological clocks do," said Knight.

One of his group's projects involves applying this type of model to identify mismatches between a person's biological and chronological age. If the biological age is notably higher, they may be unhealthy and at risk for various diseases. If it is lower, it may be possible to identify microbes that are protective factors against disease.

Knight said that ML has been used to relate the microbiome to nutrition. One study put 800 people on continuous glucose monitors and measured a variety of factors that led to individualized glycemic responses to a defined sequence of meals (Zeevi et al., 2015). This enabled the researchers to isolate the effect of different foods on postprandial blood glucose response and show that the response for a particular person to a particular food varied greatly. One surprising finding was that for a sizable fraction of the cohort, rice was worse for their blood sugar than ice cream, and the microbiome was the best predictor of who was in which group.

These findings suggest that it might be possible, said Knight, to change the microbiome to put someone into the category of people who should eat ice cream instead of rice. Addressing metabolic issues that were rare but are now more prevalent may be possible through a better understanding of how nutrition affects the microbiome and today's common chronic diseases.

Knight noted the concern about the connection between ultraprocessed foods and the increased risk for developing type 2 diabetes, cardiovascular disease, and dementia, all of which ML models have shown to be closely linked to the microbiome. To better understand this connection, his group has been looking at how the microbiome and metabolome change throughout the body under different conditions. One experiment evaluated changes in the metabolome and microbiome of mice following a single dose of one of two antibiotics (Vrbanac et al., 2020). The surprise finding, said Knight, was that the antibiotics changed molecules throughout the body, showing that a spatial understanding of changes in the body has become increasingly important for microbiome research.

His team has been collaborating with a group in Italy to study the microbiome in a village of 300 centenarians. "We are looking for factors that improve health span and lead to very long residuals from the overall microbiome and metabolome aging models," said Knight. One idea is that the bioactive compounds in rosemary somehow affect the microbiome and metabolome in a way that leads to a long life. A three-dimensional analysis of bioactive molecules in rosemary plants, measured using mass spectroscopy, found a specific spatial distribution of them throughout the plant (see Figure 3-2). This information can be useful, he said, for understanding the ethnobiology of how particular plants are used by various populations.

Knight and his collaborators launched the Global FoodOmics project to understand at the molecular level what is happening in the human body, cross-reference that to what is coming out of the body at the molecular and microbiome level as measured by the American Gut Project, and do meta-analyses to combine them. The work has provided insights into the profound transformation of foods by the microbiome as they pass through the gastrointestinal tract. Another finding has been the discovery of new bile acids produced by the microbiome with nonrandom distributions (Quinn et al., 2020). "This is an exciting direction toward understanding how microbes modify these bile acids, including with dietary components and

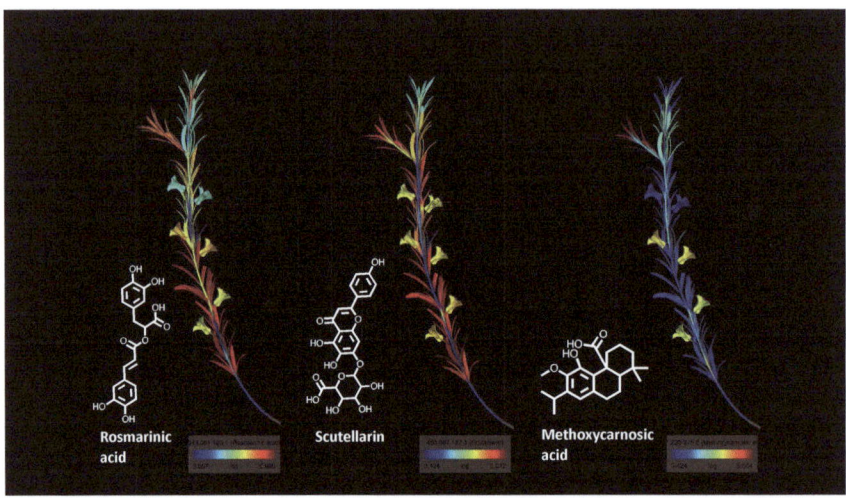

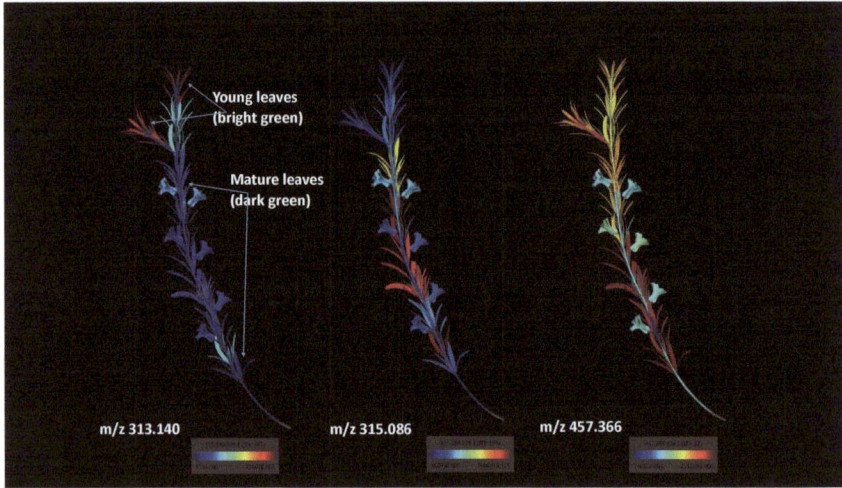

FIGURE 3-2 Distribution of known (top) and unknown (bottom) bioactive molecules in rosemary.
SOURCE: Presented by Rob Knight on October 10, 2024, at the workshop on The Role of Advanced Computation, Predictive Technologies, and Big Data Analytics in Food and Nutrition Research.

in response to them, and modify a wide range of physiological properties that are linked to different medical conditions," said Knight.

Using a new tool they developed, Greengenes2, Knight's team and their collaborators solved the problem of being unable to reconcile microbiome data collected by two different methods (McDonald et al., 2023). They also searched for specific molecules produced by the microbiome, including in mixed samples, such as stool or food (Zuffa et al., 2023). In another project, his group has been looking at the connections between the microbiome and diet in Alzheimer's disease, examining the effects of diets known to affect disease risk on microbiome and metabolome changes.

One early success from the Global FoodOmics project was demonstrating that they could read out an individual's diet directly from a biospecimen via molecular analysis (Gauglitz et al., 2022). Molecular analysis of fecal samples easily distinguished between omnivores and vegetarians, for example. Using the same technique, Knight's team is using a standardized test for verbal learning to identify particular foods that correlate with memory. Sugarcane and soda correlated with the most forgetting and worst ability to learn, and fish, strawberries, and mushrooms correlated with the best improvements in learning. A search of the literature found extensive evidence tying soda and sugar consumption to Alzheimer's risk and memory loss and supporting the idea that fish is good for preventing Alzheimer's disease and for memory in general. More limited studies have found that mushrooms and strawberries may also improve memory. "What is exciting is that with an afternoon on the mass spectrometer, we were able to recapture thousands of person-years of research across these different foods," said Knight.

Knight is involved in the Nutrition for Precision Health (NPH) component of the *All of Us* Research Program, which aims to extensively genotype and phenotype 1 million Americans. The nutrition project involves three modules. The first is a detailed characterization of 10,000 people at baseline on normal diets. The second has the participants following three crossover diets at home, and the third has 500 people on specific diets in a clinical setting. "The reason why we need these three modules is that the first module is providing the big data for ML, the second module is providing intervention data for predicting the response, and then in the third module, we'll be able to test the data with ground truth in a clinical setting," said Knight. The overall goal is to take the resulting large dataset, distill it into something that is AI ready, and use ML to predict meal response curves, uncover relationships between diet-related diseases and individual metabolic phenotypes, and identify drivers of diet- and nutrition-related health disparities.

A second goal is to engineer bacteria from an individual, reintroduce them into the gastrointestinal tract, and alter "bad" microbiomes (Russell et al., 2022). One application of this, said Knight, would be to improve cancer treatment efficacy in the two-thirds of people whose microbiomes render certain therapies ineffective. Groundbreaking research has demonstrated that dietary fiber and certain probiotics influence the gut microbiome and melanoma immunotherapy response (Spencer et al., 2021). However, this study also found that although fiber was beneficial, patients taking probiotics died earlier than those who did not. Caution is warranted, he said, in following recommendations for probiotics that have only been tested in healthy people.

Knight noted ethical considerations with microbiome interventions, particularly around bias in the training set, the ability to stratify the data, and how that stratification information is used equitably and safely. These same considerations likely apply to dietary interventions. Microbiome studies have also raised concerns about the safety of probiotics.

QUANTITATIVE ANALYSIS OF METABOLOMICS DATA TO INFORM PRECISION HEALTH

Susan McRitchie is the lead biostatistician and program manager in the Metabolomics and Exposome Laboratory at the University of North Carolina at Chapel Hill Nutrition Research Institute, and the concepts and results presented were from the Sumner Lab. She said that metabolomics is the methodology to study the low-molecular-weight complement of cells, tissues, and biological fluids. An individual's metabotype is the signature, or biochemical fingerprint, of low-molecular-weight metabolites present in tissues or biological fluids and is ideal for studying precision nutrition and precision medicine (Sumner et al., 2020). The metabolomic signature comprises endogenous metabolites reflecting host and microbial metabolism and exogenous metabolites derived from external exposures throughout an individual's life. "Metabolomics contributes to metabolic individuality because it encompasses all these complex interactions between the environment, the genome, our gut microbes, and xenobiotics," said McRitchie. "The metabolic profile shows us the biologic perturbations in host and microbial metabolism, our internal exposome, as well as our life-stage exposures."

McRitchie said that researchers frequently use metabolomic studies to discover biomarkers, including early-stage biomarkers that provide an opportunity to intervene early in the disease process and biomarkers for monitoring therapeutic response. Common biospecimens include urine, serum, and plasma, but saliva, hair, fecal samples, and breath can also provide useful data. Metabolomic studies can be hypothesis driven, to answer a specific question, or data driven, using ML to identify patterns. Researchers can use that information to design a study question. Metabolomic data can be analyzed alone or incorporated with other 'omics data.

Model systems and human subject investigations, said McRitchie, have shown that the metabotype correlates with sex, race, age, ethnicity, polymorphism, stress, weight status, mental health status, blood pressure, many disease states, the gut microbiome, diet, and physical activity. Each factor contributes to differences in levels of endogenous metabolites, which can be considered differences in internal exposure. Many chemicals, drugs, medications, and nutrients can affect the endogenous metabotype, and many can be analyzed simultaneously with host and microbial metabolites using untargeted methods. Metabolomic studies can provide mechanistic insights from pathway analysis that can identify pharmacologic targets, nutritional interventions, and genetic links to disease.

McRitchie explained that investigators acquire metabolomics data primarily from nuclear magnetic resonance or mass spectrometry, and both methods can use a variety of biospecimens. A targeted method will focus on a particular set of analytes or pathways, and an untargeted method can detect 10,000–40,000 signals. Techniques such as principal component analysis are good at reducing the dimensionality and visualization of the data. Various supervised methods can identify features important to a specific phenotype. In addition, researchers now use a variety of ML and DL methods, including random forests, neural networks, and even some deep learning models, to analyze the data.

In one study, a collaboration between the Sumner Lab and Harvard University, McRitchie used logistic regression analysis to find an early biomarker of placental abruption (PA), a rare but serious disorder of pregnancy that has no universally accepted diagnosis (Gelaye et al., 2016). The earliest but nonspecific symptoms include vaginal bleeding that occurs in some patients in the third trimester. The study's goal was to identify biomarkers from second-trimester serum that protects against PA in the third trimester. Using the Biocrates AbsoluteIDQ® p180 kit, which allows for the simultaneous quantitation of up to 188 endogenous metabolites, 9 metabolites were significantly associated with PA; they used 2 in the final model.

Logistic regression modeling for the probability of PA using vaginal bleeding in the third trimester as the predictor had an area under the curve (AUC) of 63 percent, whereas modeling with the two metabolites had an AUC of 68 percent. This was not a statistically significant increase, so it may initially seem unimportant, said McRitchie, but the key is that the latter is a second-trimester biomarker for PA in the third trimester. Further investigation into how the two metabolites are connected mechanistically to PA found that low levels of choline, known to be associated with pregnancy complications, might be a factor in PA. "It is possible that PA could be mitigated by increasing choline early in pregnancy or for women of childbearing age," said McRitchie. "This needs to be replicated in another cohort, but it is a promising result."

McRitchie briefly discussed the concept of the exposome in precision nutrition. Exposome research is key because it provides an understanding about how exposures and changes in endogenous metabolism are linked to an individual's genetics and states of health and wellness. Pathway perturbations, she said, can help identify potential targets for nutritional and pharmacologic interventions.

To conduct exposome studies, the Sumner Lab and others use mass spectrometry for untargeted analysis, and the lab uses open-source software to preprocess the data and rapid algorithms to match signals in the mass spectrum to an in-house library of over 2,500 compounds and to public databases. In addition to essential nutrients, this method detects host and microbial metabolites, environmental metabolites, drug and medication metabolites, essential nutrients, and food metabolites. Simultaneously detecting metabolites is crucial, said McRitchie, because healthy biochemistry depends on essential nutrients, which serve as cofactors for hundreds of biochemical reactions, play a role in transcription, are antioxidants, and are involved in many specialized functions. Different exposures, she added, can affect the speed of metabolism and how the body absorbs or transports nutrients and vitamins. Responders and nonresponders are important in precision nutrition, McRitchie noted, because individuals have different nutrient requirements and can have different responses to nutrient intakes. An individual's response is going to be related to their exposures, health status, and their genetics, she stated, and studying how people respond allows for discovering mechanisms and identifying nutritional targets.

One study, a collaboration among the Sumner Lab, University of Tehran, National Cancer Institute, and National Institute on Drug Abuse, aimed to find an objective marker of opium use disorder to supplement the qualitative diagnostic criteria and provide insights into mechanisms for developing intervention strategies (Ghanbari et al., 2021; Li, Y. et al., 2020). Her team analyzed urine samples from users and nonusers and found mass spectrometry signals differentiating the two groups, including perturbations in vitamins and vitamin-like compounds, neurotransmitter metabolism, Krebs cycle metabolism, glucogenesis, one carbon metabolism, lipid metabolism, and environmentally relevant metabolites. Validation of this metabolic signature might find use as an objective biological marker of opium use disorder and render it possible to develop a nutrient cocktail capable of mitigating addiction.

McRitchie discussed another study involving both metabolomics and microbiome data that aimed to identify biomarkers for and pathways involved in osteoarthritis (Loeser et al., 2022; Rushing et al., 2022). Untargeted analysis of fecal samples from individuals with obesity and with or without osteoarthritis found metabolic disruptions related to intestinal permeability, perturbations related to precursors of polyunsaturated fatty acids, such as omega-3, levels of the short-chain fatty acid propionate, which is produced by microbes in the colon and associated with dietary fiber intake, and levels of glucosamine, a component of cartilage. These findings suggest a possible nutritional intervention based on the ratio of omega-3 to omega-6 fatty acids, dietary fiber and protein, and supplementation with glucosamine and short-chain fatty acids.

A data-driven correlation analysis identified a link between osteoarthritis, gut microbes, and environmentally relevant metabolites, inflammation markers, and endogenous and microbial metabolism. One signal matched that of an insecticide associated with a particular herbicide, and others matched to compounds abundant in fruits and vegetables, suggesting that they could be the source of exposure to the herbicide. The insecticide also correlated with gut microbes from a phylum that produces short-chain fatty acids, consistent with the earlier findings.

McRitchie mentioned specialized repositories for metabolomics data, including the National Institutes of Health (NIH)-funded Metabolomics Workbench[1] that accepts both untargeted and targeted data and has publicly available data from over 2,000 studies. Several large-scale NIH consortia are also including metabolomics data, including the NPH,[2] Molecular Transducers of Physical Activity,[3] Human Health Exposure Analysis Resource,[4] Environmental Influences on Child Health Outcomes,[5] and Trans-Omics for Precision Medicine.[6] These repositories include both metabolomics data and metadata. Metadata have data privacy issues, however, and one way the consortia are dealing with this is to keep the metadata in their data center and store metabolomics data on the Metabolomics Workbench.

In addition to Metabolomics Workbench, McRitchie noted that public databases for metabolite annotations include FoodDB;[7] Phenol-Explorer, with annotations of over 500 polyphenols;[8] PhytoHub;[9] and the Human Metabolome Database,[10] with annotations for over 220,000 metabolites. Publicly available data analysis resources also include MetaboAnalyst.[11]

---

[1] Available at https://www.metabolomicsworkbench.org (accessed January 9, 2024).
[2] Available at https://www.researchallofus.org/data-tools/workbench (accessed January 9, 2024).
[3] Available at https://motrpac-data.org (accessed January 9, 2024).
[4] Available at https://hhearprogram.org/data-center (accessed January 9, 2024).
[5] Available at https://publichealth.jhu.edu/echo (accessed January 9, 2024).
[6] Available at https://topmed.nhlbi.nih.gov/topmed-data-access-scientific-community (accessed January 9, 2024).
[7] Available at https://foodb.ca (accessed January 9, 2024).
[8] Available at http://phenol-explorer.eu (accessed January 9, 2024).
[9] Available at https://phytohub.eu (accessed January 9, 2024).
[10] Available at https://hmdb.ca (accessed January 9, 2024).
[11] Available at https://www.metaboanalyst.ca (accessed January 9, 2024).

APPLICATIONS OF AI IN NUTRITION RESEARCH

Benoît Lamarche said that AI applications in nutrition research include increasing the field's capacity to manage and analyze big datasets, dietary assessment, predicting outcomes, and social media content analysis. Calling nutrition a "traditional field," he said that the challenge to realizing these applications' potential will be breaking the mold and adapting to new methods.

In the first example of an AI-based application for nutrition, Lamarche discussed a tightly controlled feeding study in which men and women with metabolic syndrome ate a North American diet for 5 weeks and then a Mediterranean diet for 4 weeks to determine the effect on the metabolome. The goal was to develop an ML algorithm that classifies people according to their diet based on untargeted metabolomics data. The resulting algorithm was 99 percent accurate, far better than the typical published study, and it showed the value of having full control of the diet, which generates a much cleaner dataset. When Lamarche and his collaborators repeated the experiment with self-reported dietary intake data, the dataset had much more noise, and the accuracy of the same ML algorithm dropped by almost 20 percent.

The lesson from this study, said Lamarche, is that the signature may not be accurate when using either untargeted or targeted metabolomics without carefully controlling the diet. This is an important issue because most of the published studies of this sort rely on self-reported dietary intake data. "It is going to be a challenge to make sense of all of this at the end of the day because we know the accuracy of these signatures in terms of predicting the right diet is going down as there is more noise in the data," he said.

Lamarche explained that for precision nutrition, the idea is to use all the data available from one individual to predict a health outcome. One study, for example, put prediabetic individuals on the Mediterranean diet or a personalized postprandial management diet based on information from microbiome data, blood tests, questionnaires, anthropometrics, and food diaries (Ben-Yacov et al., 2021). Creating the personalized diet relied on an ML algorithm that integrates these data to predict postprandial glucose responses, and the mean daily glucose levels and postprandial glucose levels were significantly lower in this group, showing that using more data to personalize the intervention was working. The challenge, said Lamarche, is figuring how to implement this type of intervention in clinical practice.

As an example of how AI can benefit precision public health, Lamarche discussed a study that characterized and mapped local environments depending on the relative proportion of low-quality food offerings to supermarkets and compared that to a map of socioeconomic status and dietary habits from Web-based dietary intake data. The ML model developed from these data could identify where people have a low-quality diet and live in a low-quality food environment. From a public health perspective, this type of mapping model can identify those areas where the environment is unfavorable to high diet quality and develop interventions that change the environment of those areas. One caution, said Lamarche, is that these maps could lead to stigmatization of different neighborhoods.

Lamarche noted that a variety of AI and ML methods can provide a better understanding of dietary patterns (see Figure 3-3). One study, for example, constructed a food network to understand meal patterns in pregnant women with high- and low-quality diets (see Figure 3-4) (Schwedhelm et al., 2021). The investigators used the Louvain community algorithm, which can detect communities in large networks to identify relationships among the different foods and communities of foods consumed together at different meals. The low-quality diet group had certain patterns of intake, such as consuming cheese more systematically with white bread.

Lamarche said that the current thinking is that AI will improve the ability to predict outcomes, although this idea is based mainly on studies with clear outcomes—disease positive versus disease negative, for example. For clear-cut outcomes, AI may indeed perform better than traditional statistical models. However, nutrition data are more "noisy," and if the outcome is a prediction of dietary intake, AI results may become murky. His group measured dietary intakes using repeated Web-based 24-hour recalls and compared the accuracy of classical logistic regression and a variety of ML methods in predicting vegetable and fruit consumption (Côté et al., 2022). Prediction accuracy for all methods, including logistic regression, was low, approximately 60 percent even with models using information from hundreds of variables. Tweaking the ML models to try to make them more appropriate for the data had little effect. In addition, the ML models and logistic regression model retained different variables. If the goal is not just to develop an accurate model but to understand which set of variables predict adequate consumption, the answer will depend on the model, which is a problem. "We tried to understand why the models were not retaining the same variables to predict the consumption of vegetables and fruit with the same accuracy, but we could not find the reason," he said.

Another example of how AI can contribute to nutrition research is exploring the relation of social media content to different food consumption patterns in different populations, said Lamarche. One study, for example, looked at tweets related to foods in Canada to assess health activity and nutritional habits (see Figure 3-5) (Shah et al., 2019). Many challenges exist to using these data, however. For example, a tweet stating that someone is a tough cookie would need to be scrubbed from the dataset, which would require a great deal of work. "When you start doing these kinds of analyses, you are going to spend 80 to 90 percent of your time cleaning the data before you can actually run something," said Lamarche.

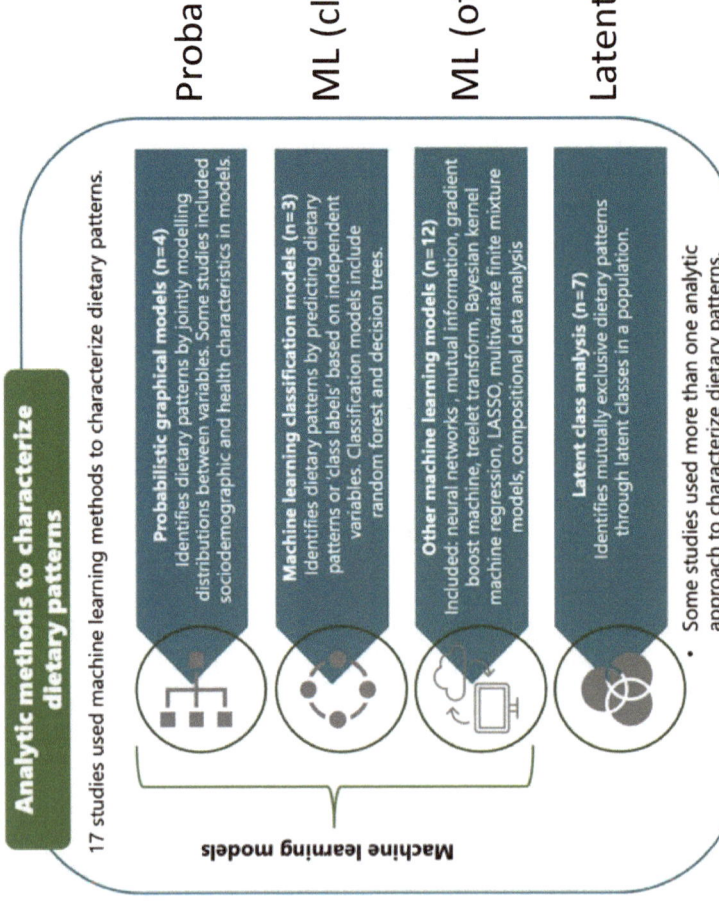

FIGURE 3-3 Analytic methods to characterize dietary patterns.
SOURCE: Presented by Benoît Lamarche on October 11, 2024, at the workshop on The Role of Advanced Computation, Predictive Technologies, and Big Data Analytics in Food and Nutrition Research. (Reprinted with Permission from Sharon Kirkpatrick.)

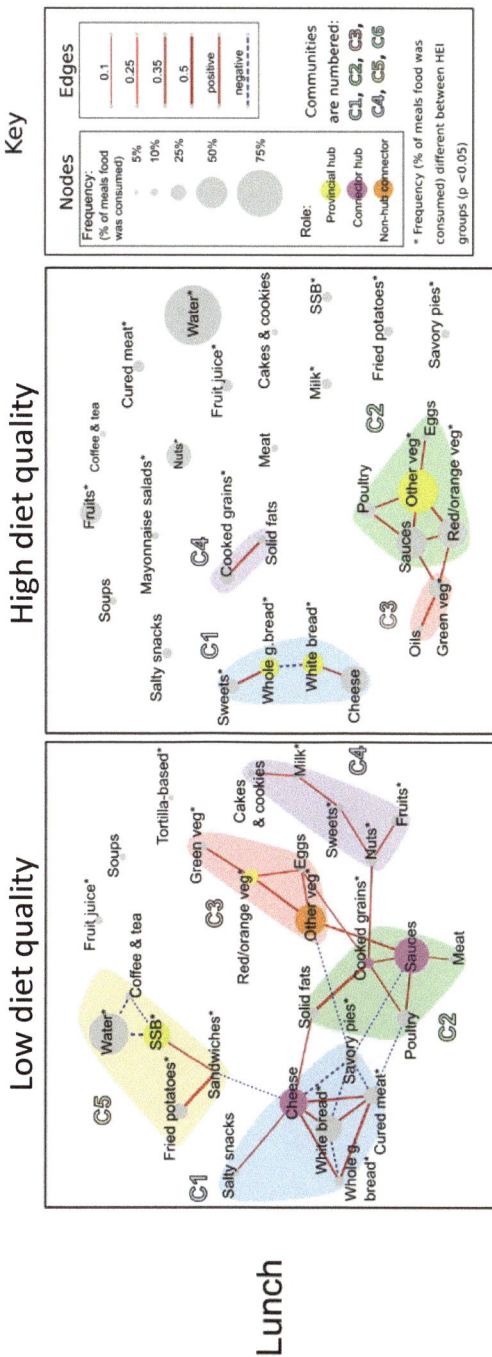

FIGURE 3-4 A food network to understand meal patterns.
SOURCE: Presented by Benoît Lamarche on October 11, 2024, at the workshop on The Role of Advanced Computation, Predictive Technologies, and Big Data Analytics in Food and Nutrition Research; Schwedhelm et al., 2021.

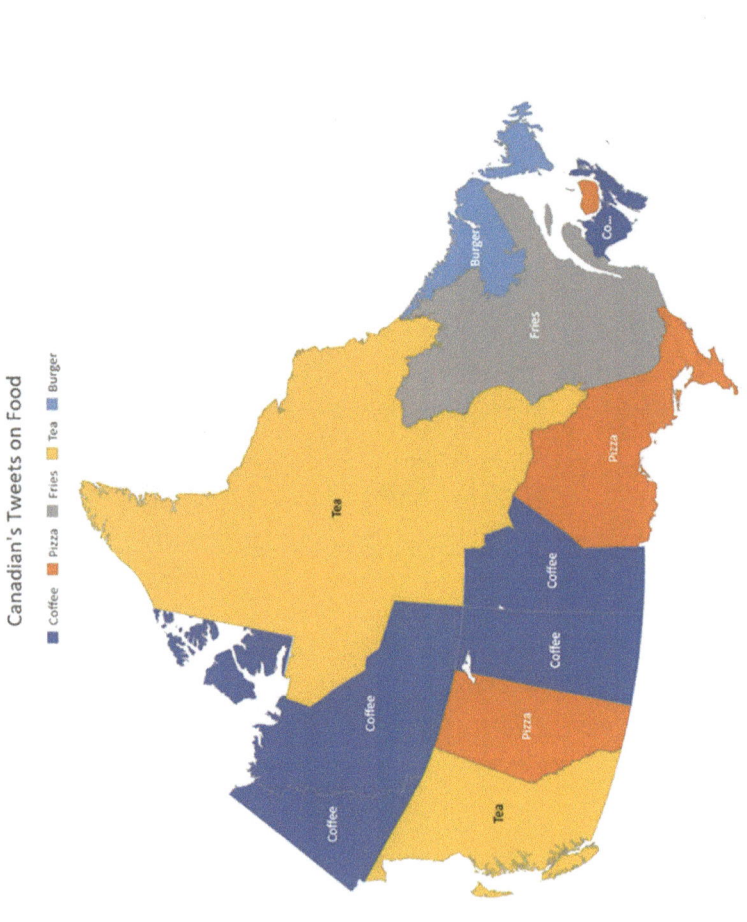

FIGURE 3-5 Natural language processing of tweets reveals geographic differences in food consumption patterns.
SOURCE: Presented by Benoît Lamarche on October 11, 2024, at the workshop on The Role of Advanced Computation, Predictive Technologies, and Big Data Analytics in Food and Nutrition Research; Shah et al., 2019.

Lamarche said that AI has great potential for the nutrition field but also significant challenges, such as appropriately considering data quality, developing a common language between nutrition and computational science, and standardizing methods and approaches. He recommended keeping an open mind about what AI can and cannot do to address what is important in nutrition.

DESIGNING NUTRITION STUDIES FOR AI DATA ANALYSIS

Sai Krupa Das, senior scientist on the Energy Metabolism Team at the Jean Mayer USDA Human Nutrition Research Center on Aging and professor at the Friedman School of Nutrition Science and Policy at Tufts University, said that the growing intersection of AI and nutrition research provides exciting opportunities for streamlining conventional research protocols and revolutionizing clinical nutrition applications. Although the size of the task can seem overwhelming, she believes it is a great time to convene to explore the opportunities. AI, she said, can be especially useful in analyzing complex data, informing adaptive study designs, and providing personalized nutrition interventions. However, these advancements come with challenges that must be addressed by multidisciplinary teams.

In Das's view, much of the difficulty in crafting personalized nutrition recommendations lies in understanding the interplay among internal (e.g., microbiome, genetics) and external factors (e.g., diet physical activity) that produce variations across individuals. Approaches are primarily in fields such as genomics, proteomics, and metabolomics, but a comprehensive understanding requires an integrated, systems-wide approach (see Figure 3-6) (Verma et al., 2018). For disease prevention, studies investigating variable responses to the same intervention also must also quantify the unique responses from people in various disease states. Nonetheless, she said, a tremendous opportunity exists to address these components and convert the challenges into real science that informs human health. "The time is certainly now. However, instead of dismissing the process as 'garbage in, garbage out,' AI inputs need to be carefully managed, and the algorithms need to be thoughtfully trained. We need to improve our methods, improve our processes, improve our workflow, and improve our infrastructure," said Das.

For nutrition scientists such as herself, the first challenge to overcome is to move away from a reductionist, hypothesis-driven approach to research design that examines singular biological pathways or outcomes. Rather, said Das, nutrition research needs to investigate the dynamic interactions between pathways that are not always linear. For example, a study of time-restricted eating and weight, stratifying early and late eaters, found no significant group difference in weight loss effectiveness (Garaulet et

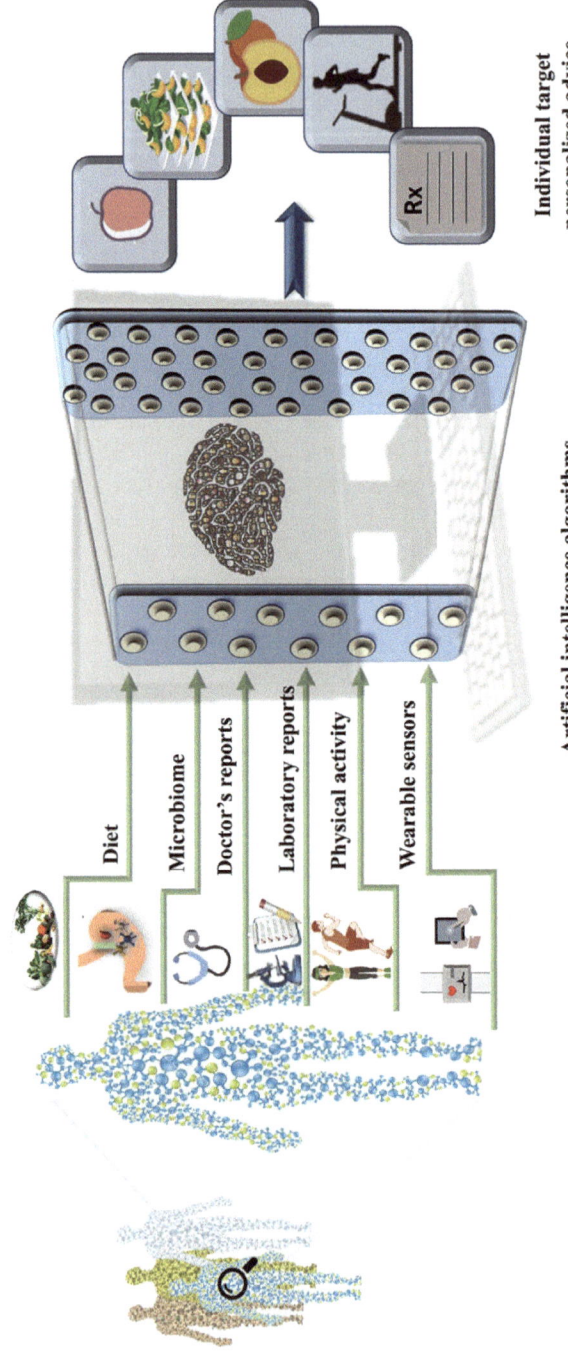

FIGURE 3-6 Solving the challenges of using AI to enable precision nutrition requires a multiscale, multisystem approach.
SOURCE: Presented by Sai Das on October 11, 2024, at the workshop on The Role of Advanced Computation, Predictive Technologies, and Big Data Analytics in Food and Nutrition Research; Verma et al., 2018.

al., 2013). However, when genetic predisposition was factored into the analysis, approximately 5 kilograms of weight loss separated individuals with one variant of the *PLIN1* gene versus another variant, suggesting the importance of multiple factors that may help explain response variability or intervention efficacy (Garaulet et al., 2016).

Das noted that over the past 2–3 decades, data have been collected on a variety of factors but that the challenge has been that such data exist in silos. "What we need is to set up study designs and infrastructure where there is multiscale input built in from the start and data integrated within one platform," said Das. Multiscale data include genetics, age, race, ethnicity, microbiome, the built environment, medication use, the biological clock, diet, medical records, and lifestyle, physiological, and social behaviors. She noted that the core requirement of a personalized nutrition computational infrastructure is that it needs to be classified and identified as a food and health infrastructure. It requires four components: the determinants of food choice, past and current intake of food and nutrients, status and functional markers of nutritional health, and health and disease risk (Snoek et al., 2018). Hard research infrastructures, or toolkits, and technical equipment for AI-powered nutrition research include applications, devices, digital health, wearable technology, digital medicine, and digital therapeutics; soft research infrastructures include telehealth or telemedicine, health information technology, and Web-based assessment using a cloud-based data source (McClung et al., 2022).

Managing and implementing the food and health infrastructure for designing studies should be user-driven, said Das, and should include the following:

- nutrition bioinformatics structures, including all biologically relevant data, preprocessed 'omics data, and descriptive and study participant phenotype data, with a priority of processing n-of-1 data;
- data management;
- data processing that includes an informatics infrastructure with standardized food intake monitoring;
- data-sharing capabilities; and
- platforms, such as web portals, for publishing the data derived from the studies to a bigger community (Verma et al., 2018).

"These are all important components in study design, and they need to be built in while the study is being designed and while the infrastructure is being put together, rather than afterward, as retrofitting these components will not work right," said Das. Establishing a food and health infrastructure for designing studies, she added, will ensure that the data related to food constituents, intake, energy expenditure, environmental variables, determinants of health, and disease risk are all in one place. These data can help elucidate the determinants of behavior that can be used to develop prediction algorithms and nutritional interventions (Verma et al., 2018).

Das listed several considerations regarding data collection when designing a study. For dietary data, these include the methodology, whether food intake diaries, 24-hour recalls, questionnaires, devices, or apps; biases in recall, reactivity, reporting, and portion size; adherence to the study protocol and related definitions, data collection, and data reporting; tools, including devices, apps, and measures or reference standards; and standardized databases that include ethnic foods and sync with other measures. Similarly, assessing physical activity has important considerations, such as how to deploy questionnaires, tracking apps, and wearables and clean and integrate the data. Considerations for biospecimen collection include biospecimen type, whether measurements are continuous or snapshots in time, specimen processing, and analysis that includes relational data and accounts for intra- and interstudy differences.

Although AI is useful for 'omics analysis, it may be important to capture all the 'omics measurements to help with phenotyping or deeply characterizing individual responses to an intervention or exposure. For example, a change may occur at the transcriptome but not the genome level and may be interpreted differently without the comprehensive measures. Das noted the importance of thinking about each input carefully when planning a study, from its design to conception to the choice of the data source and integration with the data infrastructure.

Electronic health record (EHR) data are important because they help with the human continuum from diet to wellness. However, the multiple components of an EHR contain a great deal of complexity, including sensitive information, data heterogeneity, and data structure. The benefits of digitized records include complete relational data for each person and across participants and cases, but a priori communication between AI and clinical teams is essential to ensure the data can be merged with other data collected in a study. Digitization comes with challenges such as improper standardized formats, a lack of user interface training, and poorly designed technology that leads to errors in the record. Das said that data standardization can make updating these datasets more feasible and improve communication between clinical sites. Without data standardization and harmonization, it is not possible to build a good AI-ready dataset, she added.

Das said that human studies will always have missing data, which can lead to biased and misleading results. Imputation methods can address missing data, but each method has its own drawbacks. Substituting mean or median values, for example, introduces bias for extreme values, and the K-nearest neighbors algorithm, in which values from grouped individuals can be averaged and assigned to the missing variable, may fail if individuals cannot be clearly grouped based on their clinical record values. An iterative process known as "multiple imputation by chained equations," which considers relationships between variables, is computationally intensive and assumes normally distributed data. Excluding data that are not normally distributed also can lead to bias. Das recommended consulting modelers before study implementation to establish ways of handling missing data.

An absolute must, said Das, is taking a team science approach for generating AI-ready data. Adapting to the widespread use of data-driven technologies will require supporting this approach and developing professionals with clinical and computational skills. Engaging the research team in all aspects of a project, from inception and planning to completion, analysis, and interpretation of findings, is important and will help integrate experts in all relevant fields to provide insights from diverse perspectives. Das recommended engaging data scientists as integral peer collaborators. Multidisciplinary training and education also are critical for building interdisciplinary teams, as is emphasizing that AI is a tool to inform study designs and facilitate decision making rather than a replacement for human experts.

Today, said Das, AI is informing iterative adaptive study designs (Pallmann et al., 2018). For example, a calorie restriction study might start with a meal plan. Based on a survey of preferred foods collected at baseline and analysis by an AI algorithm, researchers would then iteratively revise and customize the meal plan to maximize individual success with adherence.

Das said that the age of big data provides exciting opportunities to integrate data on food consumption and EHRs to create synthetic human cohorts that can be used to predict responses to nutrition recommendations at the system level. One primary goal for personalized nutrition, she said, is to create predictive models that draw on history of monitored health responses. The pie-in-the-sky vision, she said, is to create a geographic information system of a human (see Figure 3-7) (Topol, 2014).

AI AND THE BIG CHALLENGES IN AGRICULTURE AND FOOD

Aaron Smith, the DeLoach Professor of Agricultural Economics and lead of the AI Institute for Next-Generation Food Systems (AIFS) socioeconomics and ethics cluster at the University of California, Davis, said that the increase in agricultural productivity over the past century has been massive. In fact, U.S. farmers now produce four times as much with almost the same inputs as 100 years ago, and the world produces 250 percent more cereals on only 15 percent more land (Our World in Data, 2023; Pardey and Alston, 2021). Production, he added, has outgrown global population increase over that time.

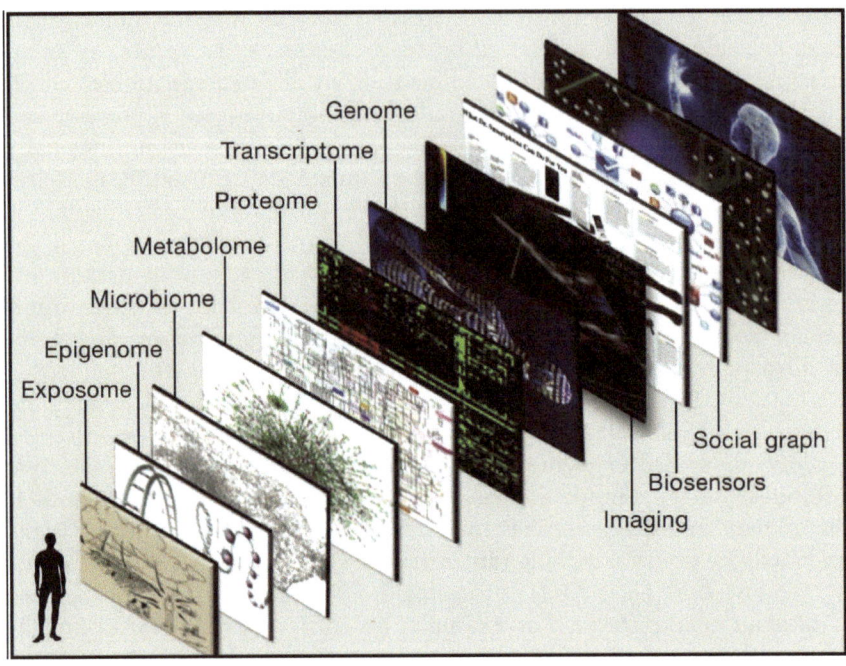

FIGURE 3-7 The layers that would make up a geographic information system of a human being.
SOURCE: Presented by Sai Das on October 11, 2024, at the workshop on The Role of Advanced Computation, Predictive Technologies, and Big Data Analytics in Food and Nutrition Research; Topol, 2014.

Smith said that higher productivity has led to lower prices, down 50 percent since 1960 on an inflation-adjusted basis. As a result, food now accounts for a much lower percentage of U.S. household budgets. Although productivity has improved the most in rich countries, the percentage of people in developing countries experiencing undernourishment has fallen by 65 percent. However, lower food prices and the availability of convenient ultraprocessed food means people eat more, resulting in over half the population in Organisation of Economic Co-operation and Development countries being overweight and nearly 25 percent obese (OECD, 2019). Over the next 30 years, these countries will spend 8.4 percent of their health budgets to treat the consequences of so many people being overweight, said Smith.

Food production is not benign, and it significantly affects the environment, said Smith (see Figure 3-8). Converting virgin land to crops, for example,

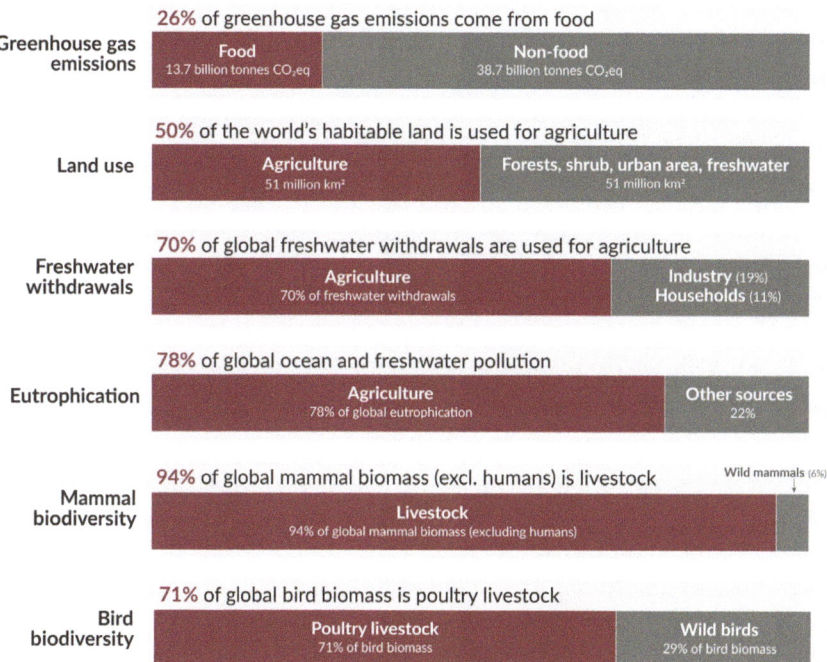

FIGURE 3-8 The environmental impacts of food and agriculture.
SOURCE: Presented by Aaron Smith on October 11, 2024, at the workshop on The Role of Advanced Computation, Predictive Technologies, and Big Data Analytics in Food and Nutrition Research; Ritchie et al., 2022.

causes massive carbon losses from soil and increased greenhouse gas emissions. Excess fertilizer application pollutes waterways, and livestock produce copious amounts of methane. Smith noted that because the global population is still increasing, food consumption will increase in the decades ahead. Perhaps more relevant, he said, is that global incomes are increasing, and as people get richer, they tend to consume more resource-intensive foods, such as beef.

One worrying sign, said Smith, is that productivity growth has slowed for the six grains responsible for the large majority of calories consumed worldwide. Continuing to increase productivity on the agricultural side is imperative to meet future calorie demands; otherwise, more virgin land will be cleared. This would exacerbate agriculture's environmental challenges.

As an economist, Smith frames this problem in terms of externalities, a side effect or consequence of an economic decision an entity makes. For example, micro-decisions in the moment about what and how much food to consume have consequences that the person's future self bears. Similarly, society bears much of the cost of health care even though individual actions largely influence one's health and thus care costs, and farmers realize the benefits of fertilizing their crops but do not bear the cost of the pollution to rivers and streams. Data are a positive externality, Smith explained, as the benefits also flow beyond the provider.

The standard Economics 101 response to externalities is to consider imposing taxes so people see the real cost of their actions when they make decisions. "I do not see any way to make that work for our food consumption decisions," said Smith, because most decisions that create these challenges are hard to change given the strong habitual element to eating and the subconscious decisions that inform eating behaviors. Although sugar taxes, for example, contribute at the margin to help people consume less sugar, manipulating human decisions by changing prices is unlikely to solve these problems, he said.

Smith said that public funding of ethical technologies to benefit society is imperative, particularly to solve problems arising from negative externalities and supercharge positive externalities. Regarding ethics and technology, he listed three core questions: who wins and who loses, who bears risk, and who decides. To Smith, the important point is that regulators' ability to constrain the development of various AI tools is limited. "It is limited by the amount of control that you have, and even if you believe that you might have a lot of control within your own country, you probably do not have control outside of your own country," said Smith.

For Smith, the ethical approach requires proactive decisions to develop technologies that would benefit society rather than focusing on regulation. "Do not pretend that by some sort of regulation and rulemaking that you are going to end up with ethical technology," said Smith. Examples of AI-enabled technologies relevant to agriculture include autonomous weeders, precision seeding and fertilizing, supply chain optimization, automatic detection of pathogens in food processing, diet customization tools, and engineering healthy foods.

When Smith and his collaborators interviewed AIFS AI researchers, the respondents expressed confidence in academic research practices and outcomes and were skeptical of the private sector, which often rushes technologies into the marketplace too quickly (Alexander et al., 2023b). The researchers commented on the complex landscape they must navigate to get data, comply with regulations, and test and deploy products. Sometimes, they reported, trustworthiness makes an AI tool less likely to be used, with the idea that it is better not to know the information that AI-generated data would reveal, such as the presence of contaminants (Alexander et al., 2023a).

Smith and his colleagues also surveyed 1,000 Illinois corn and soybean farmers to better understand their concerns about sharing data. Nearly half the farmers were unconcerned, and most of those who were concerned gave multiple reasons, including others making money off them, the top reason; an invasion of privacy; and being unsure how the data will be used. His group also asked farmers about whether they would use AI-powered technology. They voiced concerns about regulatory burdens, labor scarcity, and finance pressures. The main barriers to adoption are not related to trust issues but whether AI will solve real-life problems. "I think the same is probably true for consumers on the food side if we think about various technology tools to improve eating behaviors," said Smith.

Smith said that the priority should be to invest in problems beset by externalities and develop technologies that can help surmount the challenges of human behavior: "I think that is a much better path than trying to figure out ways to manipulate human behavior."

NOURISH OR PERISH: A RESEARCH JOURNEY THROUGH FOOD SUPPLY CHAINS

Christopher Mejía-Argueta, research scientist at the Massachusetts Institute of Technology (MIT) Center for Transportation and Logistics and founder and director of the MIT Food and Retail Operations Lab, noted that malnutrition affects other things besides health, including economic growth, social development, productivity at work, and a country's economic performance (see Figure 3-9). Moderate food insecurity affects some 1.25

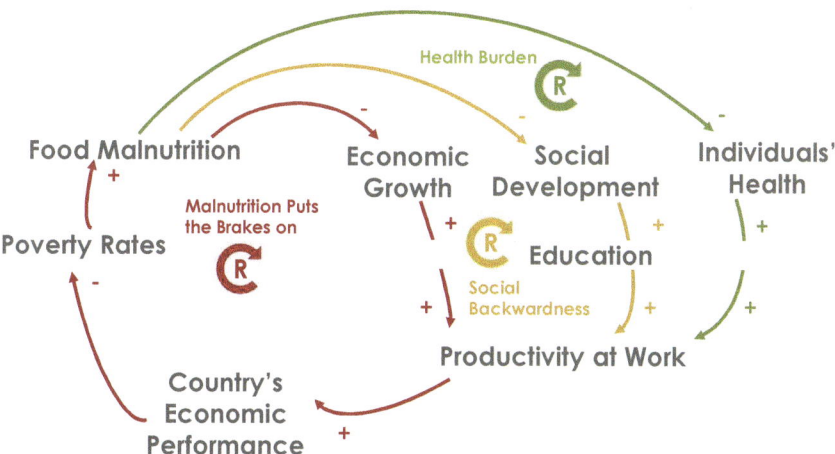

FIGURE 3-9 The widespread effects of food malnutrition.
SOURCE: Presented by Christopher Mejía-Argueta on October 11, 2024, at the workshop on The Role of Advanced Computation, Predictive Technologies, and Big Data Analytics in Food and Nutrition Research.

billion people worldwide and 143 million in Latin America and the Caribbean, and severe food insecurity affects 746 million people worldwide and 62 million people in Latin America and the Caribbean (FAO, 2020). Mejía-Argueta added that although the workshop's focus was on food, future challenges will involve water and seed availability.

Mejía-Argueta and his colleagues are tackling the challenge of malnutrition by creating innovative strategies to address the related problems of food waste or loss across the supply chain, from the field to the grocery store or farmers' market, and focusing on food safety and stakeholder behavior. He noted that technology works as an enabler, and it is important to provide good governance and policies that will be helpful for all population segments.

Supply chain management, said Mejía-Argueta, is "the systemic, strategic coordination of the traditional business functions and the tactics across these business functions within a particular company and across businesses within the supply chain, for the purposes of improving the long-term performance of the individual companies and the supply chain as a whole" (Mentzer et al., 2001). The supply chain starts with obtaining the raw materials for a product via a supplier. The manufacturer generates the product and ships it with others to a decoupling point to gain economies of scale. Usually, that point is the retailer or wholesaler, but the distributor is in charge of the decoupling. Mejía-Argueta said that the main challenge is perishability. AI and ML algorithms are embedded in the supply chain in the decision-making processes that connect the (forecasted and actual) order and inventory being managed to the consumer. AI and ML may help predict how a consumer will behave, how changes in the supply chain can affect nutrition, and how supply shocks may affect the yield and other parts of the upstream value chain.

Mejía-Argueta noted that moderately food insecure people in Latin America and the Caribbean need to pay 50 cents more per day to eat than people who are moderately food insecure in the rest of the world. Similarly, severely food insecure people in Latin America and the Caribbean pay 21 cents more per day. The reason, which also holds true in U.S. food deserts, is the negative polarity in the feedback between demand and affordability and between demand and accessibility. This dynamic makes food and vegetables expensive and hard to find and purchase for a low-income population (see Figure 3-10). For example, if a food item is too expensive to buy, shopkeepers will order less, affecting both affordability and accessibility. He noted that $3 will buy 312 calories of fruits and vegetables and nearly 3,800 calories of ultraprocessed, nonnutritious food.

The food supply, said Mejía-Argueta, is mostly inventory pushed and depends on many intermediaries (see Figure 3-11). Farmers are typically

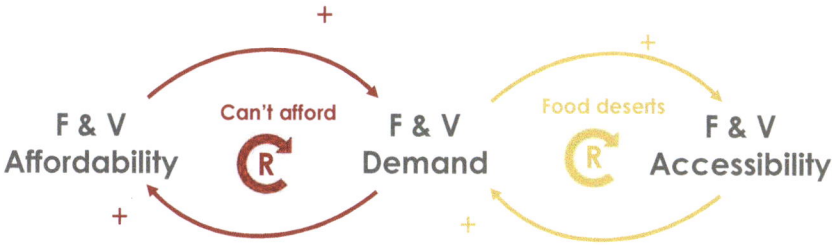

FIGURE 3-10 Negative feedback loops make fruits and vegetables expensive to eat and hard to purchase for low-income populations.
NOTE: F & V = fruit and vegetable
SOURCE: Presented by Christopher Mejía-Argueta on October 11, 2024, at the workshop on The Role of Advanced Computation, Predictive Technologies, and Big Data Analytics in Food and Nutrition Research; Sanches and Mejía-Argueta, 2019.

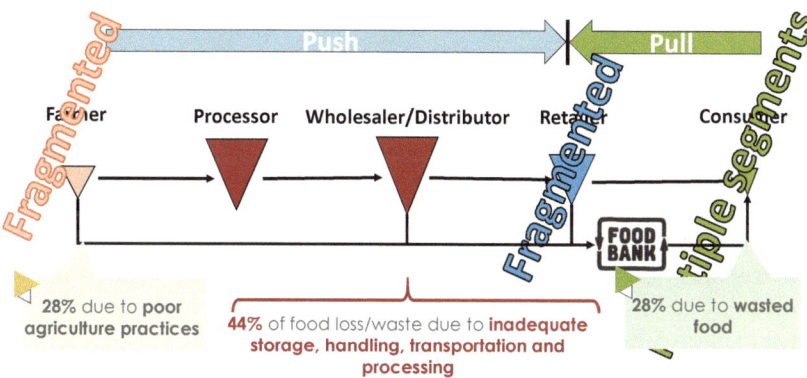

FIGURE 3-11 The current food supply chain is primarily inventory pushed and depends on a large number of intermediaries.
SOURCE: Presented by Christopher Mejía-Argueta on October 11, 2024, at the workshop on The Role of Advanced Computation, Predictive Technologies, and Big Data Analytics in Food and Nutrition Research; Sanches and Mejía-Argueta, 2019.

fragmented, particularly smallholder farmers, who account for most of the diversity in the food supply. Retailers and consumers are also fragmented. The result is that farmers account for 28 percent of food loss because of poor agricultural practices and lack of visibility, and consumers waste another 28 percent due to overpurchasing. The remaining 44 percent of food loss and waste occurs because of inadequate storage, handling, transportation, and processing.

One example of his work focused on agribusiness and involved developing an exploratory model to understand how the market size or directness to the market may affect farm gate prices. This project aimed to model how these mediators explain potato prices in Peru (Noriega et al., 2021). Mejía-Argueta noted that a big challenge, as with many modeling efforts, is having granular, high-quality data. For this study, data came from Peru's Ministry of Production and the Ministry of Agriculture, but those data do not capture what the farmers are thinking or the context around their decision-making processes. "That empathic approach is important to build the system or models from the bottom up," he said. Farmers, he added, will not use a top-down model.

The research questions Mejía-Argueta answered were to identify the factors that connect or better explain the connectivity between the market and the smallholder farmers, 80 percent of whom own less than five hectares; determine how market channel directedness or market size access affects the farm's gate price; and identify the direct or indirect influence of different factors on gate price. He explained that associativity is a critical component of market channel directness; however, it must be carefully understood to drive effective intervention schemes.

One takeaway from this project is the mixed effects on factors positively related to market directedness and negative effects on farm prices. Mejía-Argueta and his team suggest that multiple price-equilibria points exist and a geographical analysis is needed. Another lesson learned was not to overlook the importance of local demand. Larger markets do not necessarily imply higher prices, but establishing more local markets may. A further lesson was that information is not necessarily related to market accessibility or realizing a better price and that having data but possibly no real choices makes information nonactionable.

As a final example, Mejía-Argueta presented his study to increase nutrition in India by bringing more plant-based protein to the millions of people living in food insecurity whose diets lack protein, given their carbohydrate-rich diet based on rice and wheat, which the government distributes nationwide (Das, 2021). This project allowed his group to run a successful experiment to balance the production and distribution of pulses and cereals to improve the diets of each Indian state following the principle of grow local, eat healthy locally.

Elenna Dugundji, a research scientist at the MIT Center for Transportation and Logistics and a collaborator of Mejía-Argueta, briefly described several projects she has worked on with him. She discussed a project on food waste in the airline industry that combined data analytics and ML algorithms with a system dynamics framework to minimize cost and maximize the use and preservation of resources for a global airline catering company. The team also used unsupervised learning to cluster the different airports together, resulting in a more robust analysis.

Dugundji and Mejía-Argueta are investigating the effects of global supply chain disruption on U.S. food security, including whether U.S. food imports during the pandemic shifted toward being sourced over land from Latin America and/or using noncustomary maritime ports when the supply from overseas was disrupted and U.S. maritime ports were severely congested. If a shift did occur, did it persist after the pandemic ended? Another question they are studying is whether maritime ports are interchangeable in handling perishable commodities. For example, if the Port of Wilmington is disrupted, can its volume of banana imports be readily handled at a nearby port, or would this require more drastic rerouting of import flows and/or lead to food shortages at certain locations? The analysis uses a directed graph network, connecting export locations from outside the United States to import locations in the United States.

REACTION TO THE PRESENTATIONS ON APPLICATIONS AND LESSONS LEARNED

Becca Jablonski, codirector of the Food Systems Institute and associate professor at Colorado State University, noted that the potential of omitted variable bias or not considering the importance of relationships when building models are always present. She tries to deal with these by grounding conversations in the community. Regarding missing data, she called for focusing more on getting the best data possible for tipping points. The opportunity also exists to leverage unsupervised learning, especially with missing data. For her work, getting information along the supply chain is the hardest piece; good data at the farm level and decent data for the retail end of the supply chain are available, particularly for acquisition and purchasing. Supply chain data, however, are proprietary.

One of her projects is looking at the effects of policies related to food in schools and how schools respond to them. Obtaining information on what school meals look like before and after a policy goes into effect could eliminate the need for additional data collection. She also wondered about ways to use wearable technology to save time and effort required for data collection. She wants to learn more about how AI can support adaptive study designs.

Jablonski said that one of her big concerns in leading big modeling efforts is that she has not found a way to bring the best disciplinary science and robust methods to large interdisciplinary modeling projects. It is important, she said, to ensure that models reflect actual production systems in a given region. She noted that the modeling field is getting papers published in top interdisciplinary journals but not top disciplinary journals.

Regarding data, Jablonski reiterated the need to preprocess data, which requires human judgment. She noted that a lack of data can make it challenging to support historically disadvantaged and underserved farmers and ranchers without exacerbating challenges, suggesting that the federal government needs to rethink its data collection efforts. It may be fruitful, she said, for the government to invest in web scraping to get supply chain and farm gate pricing data, particularly given the growth in online platforms for farmers. Jablonski said that including behavioral components in models is important for ensuring that decision making is meaningfully integrated.

Jablonski said that the challenge in training students is balancing the trade-offs between depth and breadth. "I do not think anybody has figured out how to do this well," she said, "but this is a topic we need to think through if we want to get the topics we are talking about today right." Training students to be "T" thinkers (the vertical line is depth, and the horizontal line reflects their ability to communicate across silos) will be critical, she said, although she does not believe that pure interdisciplinary programs are the answer because students need depth in at least one area.

Jablonski's last point was about the need to show the intended beneficiaries of a model the evidence used to power it and generate ideas that can improve the end user's situation. It may be possible, she added, to use data scraping to provide data directly to U.S. Department of Agriculture (USDA), reduce farmers' data-reporting requirements, and show the end users that ML is being used to support them.

MODERATED DISCUSSION

Sharon Kirkpatrick, discussion moderator, asked the panelists for their thoughts on where the field would be in 5–10 years and about too much optimism regarding future advances. Knight replied that it is easy to both overestimate what technology will do based on extrapolations of what is possible today and underestimate how profound the changed behavior and capabilities will be, particularly if the comparison is made to other exponentially expanding technologies, such as digital photography capability or AI. Regarding possibilities such as a personal device that can analyze an individual's plate and provide them with dietary guidance, he thought that might even be possible now, but it has the ethical concern about what the device would tell the individual, how much predictive power it has, and how much of a difference the guidance would make. "The question is what can we really do [that] impact[s] health in a measurable way, has a large effect size, and is beneficial for the individual," said Knight.

Sazonov, quoting Arthur C. Clarke, said "any sufficiently advanced technology is indistinguishable from magic" and that he believes AI may become magic given the breathtaking growth of the field in recent years. Given the speed of AI development, he said that it is hard to predict where the field will be in even a few years. Lamarche predicted that, unfortunately, phone apps will tell the user what will happen if they eat a certain food but be based on unreliable data. "Someone will think about it and will invent it," he said.

When asked how federal data collection protocols could be revamped to account for cutting-edge technologies, McRitchie called for more biospecimen collection, and Sazonov wished for more information about food composition and consumption patterns. For microbiome research, Knight said that it is important to have access to original biospecimens to repeatedly analyze them with newer and better methods. He also would like to have a better understanding of how to deal with privacy issues involving reidentification associated with DNA sequencing.

Lamarche asked the panelists if they see the risk of these sophisticated analyses increasing socioeconomic disparities in health, given cost and health literacy concerns. Sazonov said that technology accessibility improves with each generation, citing that many public health interventions are designed around cell phone technology that has spread around the world. Kirkpatrick said that the struggle is whether investments should go toward developing these technologies or to addressing the social determinants of health, such as affordable housing and an affordable healthy food supply.

Knight commented that an effective method of being equitable will be to integrate analytical methods with devices people will purchase and have with them anyway, such as a cell phone camera. He also said that to mitigate disparities, it is important to design technology to avoid financial or cultural barriers. He noted that the Study of Latinos project is collecting microbiome and metabolic data and reaching out to that underrepresented demographic. Other similar projects take the *All of Us* approach to diversity, but he called for complementing that approach with studies that contact particular populations with community representatives and investigating cultural factors that can be barriers to access. McRitchie said that it will be important to work with community leaders and others who serve vulnerable populations.

A participant asked if measurement error in metabolome and microbiome assays is negligible enough that AI-generated results will be more robust than they would be with imaging data. Knight said that different analytical methods for reading the microbiome have provided markedly different results, making cross-validation and assay standardization important, but funding for standardization and quality control efforts has been limited. Microbiome assays are getting better at reproducibility regarding repeated readouts from the same biospecimen, but problems remain with things such as misalignment of readouts. He also noted the challenge of comparing data generated by different analytical methods. McRitchie said that one of the big challenges with metabolomics is that many of the metabolites seen in spectral data are unknown. Characterizing those unknowns is important because then it will be possible to develop targeted assays that provide actual concentrations as opposed to the relative amounts obtained from untargeted data.

Rodolphe Barrangou asked about a future in which models use individual genetic data and, if so, how dealing with personalized and private information will be handled. Holly Nicastro, program director in the NIH Office of Nutrition Research and program coordinator for NPH, powered by the *All of Us* research program, said that genomics will play a role in NPH, but it is unclear if individual genes or genetic markers will be predictors. "I think it would be naive to think that there would not be information to be gleaned from certain aspects of the genome and how a patient might want to eat to improve their health," said Nicastro.

Kirkpatrick asked the panelists for advice for investigators who are starting to integrate AI and data science. Knight noted the room for responsible, far-reaching technology development that encourages people to try things and discover what is possible without too many preconceived notions while having safeguards for how the results will be applied clinically. "I would say take a two-pronged approach where, on the one hand, you do not want to inhibit researchers' and especially students' creativity in trying out new and untested methods on big data, but at the same time, you want to teach them on well-understood and well-established datasets what the guardrails are for drawing correct versus incorrect conclusions," said Knight.

McRitchie suggested developing tutorials written in accessible language that identify limitations of the different methods, how to properly use a method, and how big a sample is necessary. Nicastro reiterated the importance of having study participants as partners involved in the study design and the questions they would like answered.

Barrangou commented that several speakers noted the gap between nutrition scientists and data scientists, but after listening to the presentations, he believes the relevant analogy is a mosaic. "Within nutrition, we have researchers, clinicians, food scientists, and many different kinds of sciences and disciplines, and on the AI side, we have engineers, mathematicians, data scientists, programmers, and statisticians," he said. He asked the panelists for their thoughts on what the mosaic is missing most and how to fill these gaps. Das replied that addressing the scope of AI and ML projects requires a multidisciplinary approach involving all research areas and creating a transdisciplinary approach requires awareness and the resources to support it.

Regarding data availability, Dugundji noted that USDA has dashboards showing how long trucks are waiting at different places and that the U.S. Department of Transportation convened a group of private sector parties representing different links in the supply chain to map out the data needed from each link to improve the efficiency of each step. The beneficiaries of this effort have been cargo ship owners, but she hoped the focus would include food.

Regarding training, Dugundji said that it is important that every student coming through her program graduates knowing how to program and have a basic understanding of these models so they can engage as managers of teams they may be supporting. Smith said that his institute's leadership worked hard to bring together engineers and computer scientists with domain experts for specific projects. For example, staff members are using ML tools to help researchers involved in seed development build traits in crops that will lead to tastier food, improve supply chains, and map the connections between food, micronutrients, and human health. This approach, Smith said, seems to work well, although the biggest gap is in how human behavior affects what people eat.

Mejía-Argueta agreed with these comments and added that missing pieces include strategies to be more collaborative and, from the country perspective, understand the scenario planning needed to create better and more resilient supply chains. He noted that the Netherlands creates working groups with representatives from the private sector, nonprofit organizations, government, and academia who try to understand how to prepare for future challenges in different areas. "Perhaps that is something that we should start doing, because at the end, that is probably one of the ways in which we can boost the use of all the knowledge that we have," said Mejía-Argueta. For him, one of the biggest challenges is to create the proper environment to start collaborating with each other so each collaborator gets the best of the available knowledge, awareness, techniques, and data.

Regarding how to get researchers to understand the value of moving out of their silos and be willing to share data and even work together before starting a project to increase data usability, Jablonski said that the first step is to ensure that data are generated more usably for a broader group of researchers across departments and agencies. When she conducts trainings for a variety of groups, she usually hears about the data her audience intends to collect, but they do not start with what is already available and which gaps exist. "If we do not start by understanding the data, we are going to continue to oversurvey groups and see declining response rates because groups do not see that the data they already provided are being used," she said. She noted that in response to 9/11, the federal government collected a great deal of information about the supply chain but did not make those data available across federal agencies.

Smith agreed that a great deal of data, particularly at the federal level, is hard to access. For example, USDA has data on today's price of spinach in St. Louis, but it is difficult to see how it has varied over time because those data are not stored, displayed, or made easily accessible. With his students, he has tried to build a resource catalog that lists where to find various datasets, but even that is a challenge. He noted that USDA is trying to break down silos between different parts of the department to improve data access.

According to Smith, researchers have become more willing to be transparent about their data, which is important for replicability and having trust in research products. Accessing data from private entities, including farmers and consumers, continues to be a challenge because of issues of ownership and who will profit from the information they provide. He wondered about a way to construct data agreements so that the provider benefits and the data become more accessible for projects that would improve societal outcomes.

Benoît Lamarche mentioned countries that have been successful in collecting, managing, and exploiting their data. For example, all health care data in Sweden are available to all researchers in the country. Creating such a policy of making all national data accessible requires political will, he added. In Canada, data are standardized but not accessible, with no political will to use the treasure trove of data to improve the country's systems. Dugundji said that the key to getting entities to share their data is to show them the benefits for them and create a safe haven for doing so. For example, the federal Confidential Information Production and Statistical Efficiency Act blocks efforts to subpoena any data provided to a federal agency.

Barrangou asked the panelists to opine on what they think should happen in the field over the next 3–5 years. Lamarche replied that training will be key to moving the field forward. "We need more people who are bilingual and can speak nutrition and data science," he said. Another challenge is convincing the AI community to be excited about the role it can play in social innovation and public health. Das emphasized the importance of gaining better understanding of the signal-to-noise ratio in data and the inputs that would yield a better return of investment for AI applications. She also noted that it would be important to understand the difference between interpretability and explainability when examining model produced outputs.

Smith said that the public's skepticism about nutritional information is a challenge resulting from the constantly changing advice in the popular media and the effect that has on changing food consumption patterns. Diana Thomas, professor of mathematics at the U.S. Military Academy at West Point, said that the U.S. Army has, over the past 10 years, trained some 20,000 data scientists who are eager to tackle problems relating to human performance and nutrition problems. "If you are interested in a project that you do not have time for right now but would make a yearlong project for a cadet, we have some superb cadets that could attack some of these problems that you are interested in," said Thomas.

4

Capacity Building

> **Highlights from the Presentations of Individual Speakers**[a]
> - Precision nutrition is a framework for incorporating genetics, dietary habits and eating patterns, circadian rhythms, health status, socioeconomic and psychosocial characteristics, food environments, physical activity, and the microbiome in assessing nutrition status and developing interventions. (Mehta)
> - AI could both exacerbate disparities and not close the gap for the many U.S. subpopulations experiencing higher rates of diet-related morbidity and mortality than the general population. (Odoms-Young)
> - Diversity in AI research teams is important because extensive evidence indicates that diverse teams can generate more inclusive and relevant research questions, which is important when considering the social and structural drivers that exist and link to diet-related conditions and behaviors. (Odoms-Young)
> - Trust becomes important when considering diversity and representativeness of datasets used in training AI algorithms and participation in studies, which is why it is important to include stakeholder engagement when building diverse teams and that the people engaged in studies realize the promise of that research. (Odoms-Young)

- When thinking about diversity, equity, inclusion (DEI), and belonging, intersectionality is important because all people, even those within certain subgroups, may not be the same, depending on their intersectional identities and exposure to intersectional oppression. (Odoms-Young)

[a] This list is the rapporteurs' summary of points made by the individual speakers identified, and the statements have not been endorsed or verified by the National Academies of Sciences, Engineering, and Medicine. They are not intended to reflect a consensus among workshop participants.

TRAINING PROGRAM IN AI AND PRECISION NUTRITION

Saurabh Mehta, the Janet and Gordon Lankton Professor, director of the Program in International Nutrition, founding director of the Cornell Center for Precision Nutrition and Health, and codirector of the National Institutes of Health (NIH)-funded Cornell Center for Point-of-Care Diagnostics for Nutrition, Infection, and Cancer, commented that food prevents and can be a major contributor to managing disease, but the diet–disease relationship is complex, with many endogenous and exogenous factors contributing to risk. Moreover, everyone responds differently to food. He noted that the 2020–2030 Strategic Plan for NIH Nutrition Research[1] states that precision nutrition is a unifying and holistic approach to developing comprehensive and dynamic nutritional recommendations relevant to both individual and population health. It is also a framework for incorporating genetics, dietary habits and eating patterns, circadian rhythms, health status, socioeconomic and psychosocial characteristics, food environments, physical activity, and the microbiome in assessing nutrition status and developing interventions.

Artificial intelligence (AI) will play a key role in precision nutrition because of the complexity and amount of data needed for examining the body's response to internal and external factors (see Figure 4-1) (Lee et al., 2022). These relationships, said Mehta, are further complicated by the time lag and relevant biological period when considering diet as an exposure and chronic disease as an outcome. The feedback loops omnipresent in biological systems makes the challenge of developing precision medicine even more complex.

Mehta pointed out that advanced training in AI for precision medicine is one component of building capacity. To promote that, NIH issued a request

---

[1] Available at https://dpcpsi.nih.gov/onr/strategic-plan (accessed January 9, 2024).

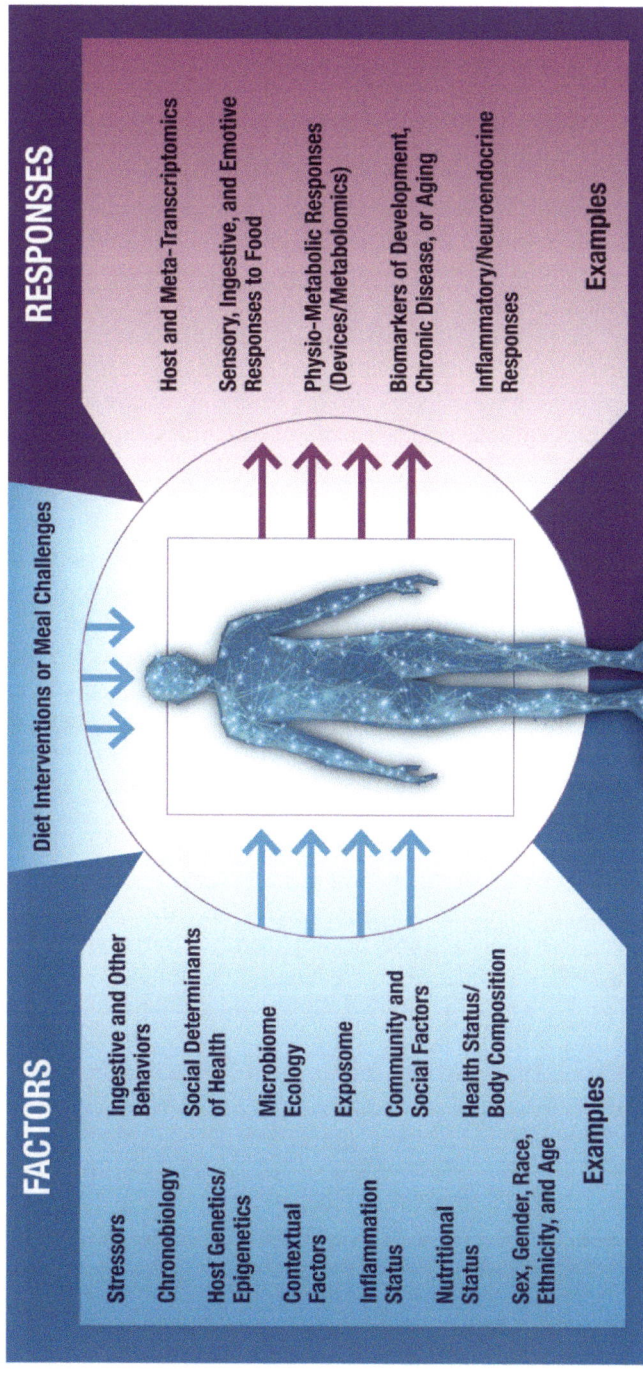

FIGURE 4-1 Factors associated with the variability between individuals in response to diet.
SOURCE: Presented by Saurabh Mehta on October 10, 2024, at the workshop on The Role of Advanced Computation, Predictive Technologies, and Big Data Analytics in Food and Nutrition Research; Lee et al., 2022.

for applications (RFA)[2] aimed at building a future workforce capable of making pivotal discoveries using an increasingly complex landscape of big data and an array of data tools to tackle complex biomedical challenges in nutrition science and diet-related chronic diseases. One RFA element called for assembling teams of interdisciplinary scientists across nutrition, biomedicine, behavioral science, and computational methods. NIH's portfolio analysis found that out of almost 2,000 NIH training grants, only 20 focused on nutrition and 28 on bioinformatics or data science.

Pulling together collaborators from four institutions at Cornell, Cornell Tech, Weill Cornell Medicine, and the U.S. Military Academy at West Point, Mehta succeeded in applying for this training grant and establishing the Cornell University Training Program in AI and Precision Nutrition.[3] Its goal is to train the next generation of scientists and build a workforce equipped with expertise in AI and ML methods to tackle complex biomedical challenges in nutrition and health using high-dimensional data. The focus, said Mehta, is applying precision nutrition to address challenges in maternal and child health.

The training program has one director and six codirectors with 23 faculty members spread across nutrition, computational biology, neurobiology, medicine, population health sciences, computer and information science, and engineering, in order to maximize the faculty and recruitment pool and provide adequate support to trainees. The program plans to add a faculty member with expertise in ethics and fairness in AI. Mehta noted the fortuitous timing because it coincided with the inception of the Cornell Center for Precision Nutrition and Health, which has three hubs: AI & Precision Nutrition, Evidence Synthesis, and Training & External Partnerships; these can serve as a home base for trainees focused on similar areas. The center can also provide supplemental funding for trainees, particularly postdocs, and provide an umbrella for bringing interdisciplinary faculty expertise together. The program will benefit from an initiative at Cornell that is building core AI capabilities and technology for human engagement.

The plan, said Mehta, is to have four predoctoral trainees and one postdoctoral trainee. The predoctoral trainees will be divided between those going for the Ph.D. in nutrition or a related biomedical field who will minor in computer science and those going for a Ph.D. in computer science who will minor in nutrition. He anticipates that the postdoctoral fellow will already have training in computational fields and want to apply that skill set to problems related to nutrition. A key aspect to this T32 program is that it will require all five trainees to have two mentors, one focused on

---

[2] Available at https://grants.nih.gov/grants/guide/rfa-files/RFA-OD-22-027.html (accessed January 9, 2024).

[3] Available at https://www.cpnh.cornell.edu/t32 (accessed January 9, 2024).

nutrition-related issues and the other on AI/computational methods, and complete a capstone course that provides them with real data to analyze. Mehta said that if the program is renewed after its initial 5 years, the goal would be to add a second postdoc with expertise in nutrition who wants to learn to apply computational techniques to nutrition research.

Mehta listed several challenges in developing this training program, starting with the need for flexibility and constant evolution. A major challenge is that computer science courses can present a steep learning curve for many nutrition Ph.D. students. The initial group of fellows may need to lean toward those with quantitative or computational backgrounds. Coursework will need to be supplemented with cocurricular activities to develop interdisciplinary scientists. This will include landscape analyses of, for example, New York City AI startups and their partners at Cornell Tech and arranging practicums, practical experiences, and needs assessment exercises with some of these partners. This T32 program may need to be more flexible in appointing trainees earlier, before their qualifying exam, to allow for full development of a truly comentored research and training plan. Mehta said that responsible conduct-of-research training will need to be reimagined and strengthened to account for ethics, fairness, and equity in AI. "This is still a program being built from the ground up," said Mehta, "and any suggestions and input are definitely welcome."

BUILDING INCLUSIVE TEAMS FOR FOOD AND NUTRITION RESEARCH

Angela Odoms-Young, the Nancy Schlegel Meinig Associate Professor of Maternal and Child Nutrition and director of the Food and Nutrition Education in Communities Program and New York State's Expanded Food and Nutrition Education Program at Cornell University, said that her remarks would focus on two key areas regarding diversity, equity, and inclusion (DEI) and belonging (see Figure 4-2):

- What is the significance of promoting diversity, equity, and inclusion (DEI), along with justice and belonging, in applying advanced computation, big data analytics, and high-performance computing in food systems and nutrition research?
- How to create a just, diverse, inclusive, and equitable training environment to support robust and ethical application of advanced computation, big data analytics, and high-performance computing in food and nutrition research?

She noted that AI could both exacerbate disparities and not be effective at closing the gaps for the many U.S. subpopulations experiencing higher

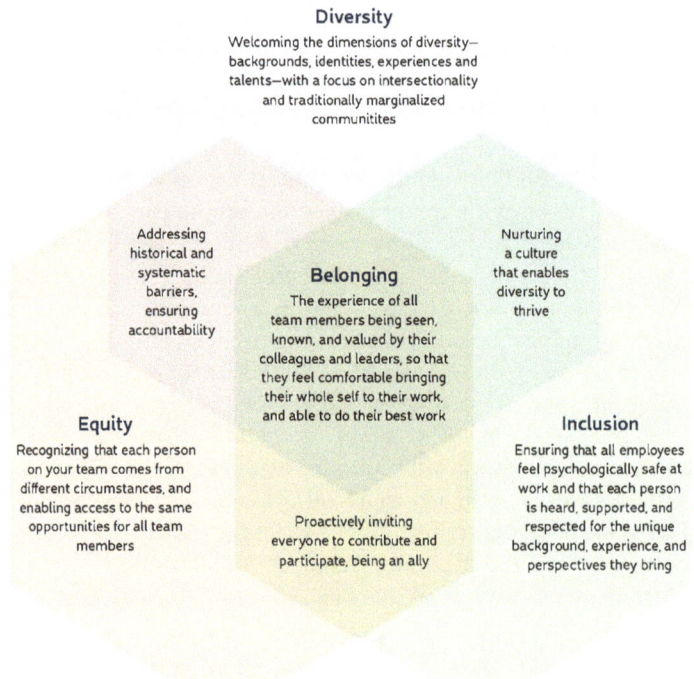

FIGURE 4-2 The overlap of DEI and belonging.
NOTE: DEI = diversity, equity, and inclusion.
SOURCE: Presented by Angela Odoms-Young on October 10, 2024, at the workshop on The Role of Advanced Computation, Predictive Technologies, and Big Data Analytics in Food and Nutrition Research. Reprinted with permission from Blue Beyond Consulting, https://www.bluebeyondconsulting.com/blog/dei-in-the-workplace-infographic (accessed January 9, 2024).

rates of diet-related morbidity and mortality than the general population (Brown et al., 2022). Although much of the work in this area focuses on race, sex, and income, similar disparities in health outcomes exist for members of the LGBTQ+ community[4] and individuals with disabilities. Despite strong efforts at the national, state, and local levels, disparities in food

---

[4] An initialism that refers to individuals, topics, and communities who are lesbian, gay, bisexual, transgender, queer/questioning. The + symbol acknowledges that there may be sexual/gender identities not represented in the other terms.

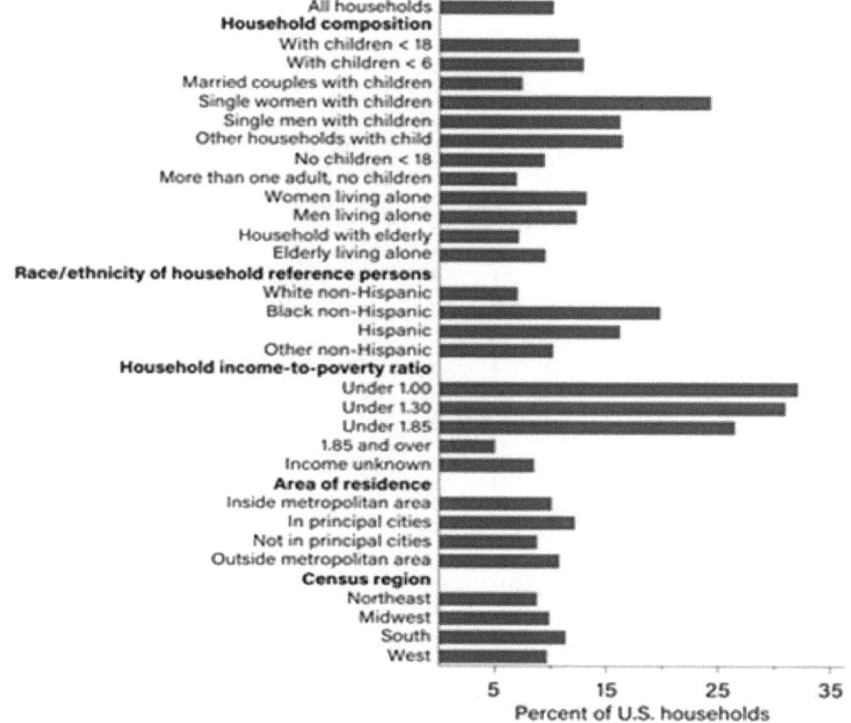

FIGURE 4-3 Prevalence of food insecurity by selected household characteristics, 2021.
SOURCE: Presented by Angela Odoms-Young on October 10, 2024, at the workshop on The Role of Advanced Computation, Predictive Technologies, and Big Data Analytics in Food and Nutrition Research; Coleman-Jensen et al., 2022.

insecurity and related outcomes continue to persist, said Odoms-Young (see Figure 4-3) (Coleman-Jensen et al., 2022).

Odoms-Young provided an example of how African American researchers could bring a different lens to nutrition research and incorporate their lived experiences with the burden of obesity in the African American population (see Figure 4-4). She said that a similar conversation has been happening within the AI field, not just in nutrition, though the two conversations are occurring in their own spheres. She quoted Timnit Gebru, cofounder of Black in AI and a member of Microsoft's Fairness, Accountability, Transparency, and Ethics in AI group: "There is a bias to what kinds of problems we think are important, what kinds of research we think are important, and where we think AI should go. If we do not have diversity in

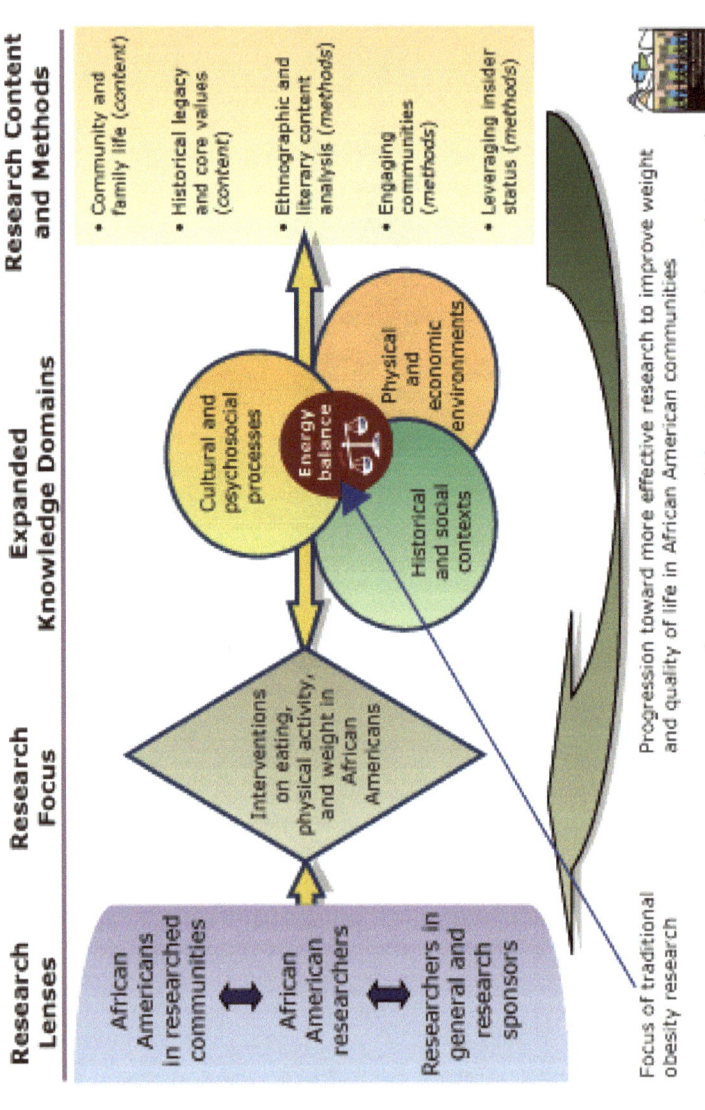

FIGURE 4-4 Bringing the perspective of African American researchers to the problem of excess obesity in African American populations.
SOURCE: Presented by Angela Odoms-Young on October 10, 2024, at the workshop on The Role of Advanced Computation, Predictive Technologies, and Big Data Analytics in Food and Nutrition Research; Kumanyika et al., 2007.

our set of researchers, we are not going to address problems that are faced by the majority of people in the world. When problems don't affect us, we don't think they're that important, and we might not even know what these problems are, because we're not interacting with the people who are experiencing them."[5]

Diversity in AI research teams is important, said Odoms-Young, because extensive evidence indicates diverse teams can generate more inclusive and relevant research questions, which is important when considering the social and structural drivers that link to diet-related conditions and behaviors (Lorenzo et al., 2017; Rock and Grant, 2016; Wegge et al., 2012; Yang et al., 2022). These diverse perspectives can enhance problem identification, decision making, and problem solving. Diverse research teams can alter the behavior of a group's social majority in ways that lead to improved and more accurate group thinking and are less likely to be influenced by unconscious biases and stereotyping, leading to more objective and unbiased findings. Diverse team members can bring unique knowledge, skill sets, and subject-matter expertise, which can enrich the process and result in a more comprehensive understanding of the subject matter. In addition, their research is more likely to reach and resonate with a broader audience based on its relevance to various communities and stakeholders.

As speakers noted, biased algorithms can create unfair outcomes that unjustifiably and arbitrarily privilege a certain group. This is important, said Odoms-Young, in that different algorithms can act as gatekeepers to health or economic opportunities. Trust, she said, becomes important when considering the diversity and representativeness of AI training datasets and study participation, which is why it is important to include stakeholder engagement when building diverse teams and that study participants realize the promise of that research.

Indigenous knowledge can offer a different way of considering how AI and people relate to one another (Williams and Shipley, 2021). AI, said Odoms-Young, encompasses a wide variety of tools and technologies that model human learning and decision making with wisdom, and wisdom is linked to worldviews. Diverse teams can bring a different worldview that helps when considering how to apply tools from different perspectives.

Odoms-Young cited numerous barriers to DEI and belonging. One barrier is implicit bias. Researchers and team leaders may have unconscious biases that influence their decision making regarding team composition and lead to underrepresentation in research teams, even when qualified candidates are available. A second barrier is limited networking opportuni-

---

[5] Available at https://www.technologyreview.com/2018/02/14/145462/were-in-a-diversity-crisis-black-in-ais-founder-on-whats-poisoning-the-algorithms-in-our (accessed January 9, 2024).

ties. Access to professional networks and mentorship is crucial for career advancement in research.

Lack of inclusive hiring practices can perpetuate a lack of representation on research teams, with traditional hiring methods potentially favoring candidates from majority groups, and tokenism, said Odoms-Young, can lead to feelings of isolation and marginalization and limit the potential impact of diverse perspectives. Experiences of microaggressions and discrimination within research teams, the fifth barrier, can create hostile work environments affecting members' well-being and professional development. Other barriers include the following:

- Inequitable allocation of resources: Individuals may face disparities in access to funding, equipment, and other necessary resources. This can hinder their ability to conduct research and publish their findings.
- Lack of representation in leadership roles: A lack of diversity among team leaders and principal investigators (PIs) can limit opportunities for career advancement and an inclusive voice.
- Culturally insensitive environments: Research teams that do not consider the cultural backgrounds and needs of individual members may inadvertently create environments that are less welcoming and inclusive.
- Limited role models: A lack of visible role models from various backgrounds can make it harder for aspiring researchers to envision successful career paths in academia or the scientific community.
- Stereotypes and preconceptions: Stereotypes about the abilities and interests of researchers can influence team dynamics and opportunities for advancement. Preconceived notions about researchers' areas of expertise may limit their involvement in certain projects.

Structural barriers also start earlier than graduate school, she noted, and breaking down those barriers should start at the high school or elementary school level.

What is striking, said Odoms-Young, is the degree of underrepresentation of minoritized populations among full-time faculty at degree-granting postsecondary institutions; in 2018, they accounted for only about 25 percent of all faculty of all ranks (Hussar et al., 2020). A similar situation is apparent when examining the percentage of doctorates conferred in science, technology, engineering, and mathematics (STEM) fields by race and ethnicity (Hussar et al., 2020). These disparities, she noted, link to funding, where African American biomedical scientists, for example, have a lower rate of NIH funding compared to White scientists (Hoppe et al., 2019). Funding, she added, is important for team diversity and an individual's sustainability in academia.

A National Science Foundation analysis found that female scientists leave the field for different reasons depending on race (Metcalf et al., 2018). Native Hawaiian and Pacific Islander women primarily leave for family, but job availability is the main reason for Black and Alaska Native women. She cited another survey of over 25,000 STEM professionals that found that, compared to non-LGBTQ+ scientists, LGBTQ+ scientists were less likely to report opportunities to develop their skills and access to the resources required to do their jobs well (Cech and Waidzunas, 2021), 20 percent more likely to have experienced some professional devaluation, such as being treated as less skilled than their colleagues, and 30 percent more likely to have experienced harassment at work in the past year. Results from the same survey suggest that LGBTQ+ scientists experience some health problems more often than their non-LGBTQ+ peers because of high levels of stress at work, microaggressions, and systemic, ongoing harassment and discrimination.

Racial gaps in net worth continue to persist, said Odoms-Young, and that can contribute to disparities in student loan debt and educational opportunities (Perry et al., 2021). In 2019, 74 percent of Black individuals with student loans had a current balance that exceeded the original loan (Perry et al., 2021), and educational attainment varies geographically, with fewer students in the South achieving a B.A. or higher compared to all other regions of the nation.

Odoms-Young said that when thinking about DEI and belonging, intersectionality is important because all people, even those within certain subgroups, may not be the same depending on their intersectional identities and exposure to intersectional oppression. She highlighted a paper on how NIH is working to foster inclusive excellence for women (see Figure 4-5) (Ten Hagen et al., 2022) and noted strategies for increasing DEI, belonging, and justice from the Nutrition Obesity Research Center (Martin et al., 2023):

- Improving outreach and recruitment by partnering with historically Black colleges and universities, Hispanic-serving institutions, and tribal colleges, and developing position descriptions that communicate an institutional commitment to DEI
- Focusing on policies, procedures, and people by guiding committee members on how to evaluate DEI in candidates, tracking data on recruitment and retention of underrepresented scientists, and evaluating to identify points of attrition contributing factors
- Creating an inclusive environment by conducting institution-wide cultural safety training, cultural and structural competence, and implicit bias training

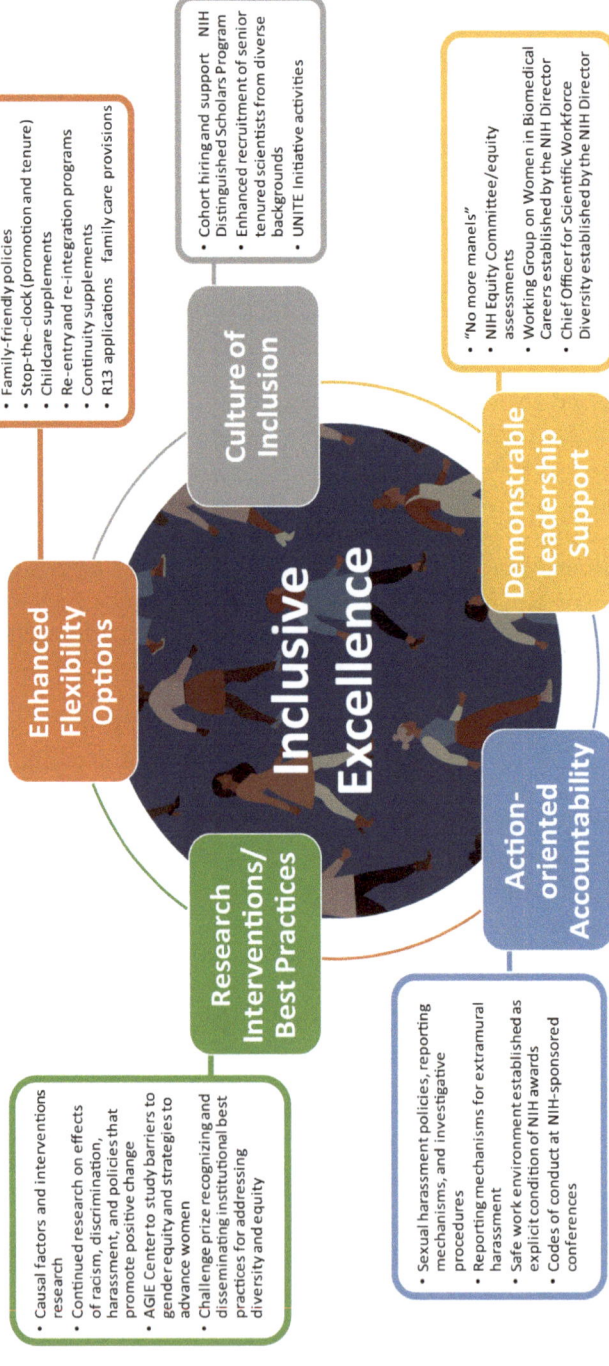

FIGURE 4-5 Move toward inclusive excellence by promoting and supporting women in science.
SOURCE: Presented by Angela Odoms-Young on October 10, 2024, at the workshop on The Role of Advanced Computation, Predictive Technologies, and Big Data Analytics in Food and Nutrition Research; Ten Hagen et al., 2022.

- Assembling diverse research teams
- Identifying and removing institutional or systemic barriers through pilot funding and equitable workloads
- Supporting community engagement
- Fostering representation in leadership
- Allowing for diverse research topics
- Evaluating progress

Odoms-Young advises her graduate students to try to implement the world they want to see. This may take time, because it requires a culture shift and for someone to emphasize the need to build diverse research teams. This shift will require people in power to make room for others; collecting data, tracking, and commitment to change; and cross-cultural mentoring to address the needs of students from diverse backgrounds that are not represented on the faculty. "There has to be some intentionality," she said, noting that equity is everyone's responsibility, not just that of people of color, LGBTQ+ people, or people with disabilities.

Odoms-Young concluded with a quote from Justice Ketanji Brown Jackson on the recent Supreme Court ruling on affirmative action:

> *Gulf-sized race-based gaps exist with respect to the health, wealth, and well-being of American citizens. They were created in the distant past, but have indisputably been passed down to the present day through the generations. Every moment these gaps persist is a moment in which this great country falls short of actualizing one of its foundational principles—the 'self-evident' truth that all of us are created equal.*

> *Our country has never been colorblind. Given the lengthy history of state-sponsored race-based preferences in America, to say that anyone is now victimized if a college considers whether that legacy of discrimination has unequally advantaged its applicants fails to acknowledge the well-documented 'intergenerational transmission of inequality' that still plagues our citizenry.*[6]

MODERATED DISCUSSION

When asked for ideas on how to train future leaders and researchers in the soft skills critical in making teams inclusive, supportive of all members, and safe from microaggressions, Mehta replied that intentionality in both formal training and in how research teams conduct themselves and interact with one another is key. Odoms-Young said that DEI training that involves

---

[6] Available at https://www.supremecourt.gov/opinions/22pdf/20-1199_hgdj.pdf (accessed January 9, 2024).

people bringing their lived experiences is paramount. It can help people realize they have the will but not the tools to be inclusive and create an environment of cultural safety. It is important to bring in a diverse set of trainees to prompt constant thinking about DEI and have empowered and inspiring trainers. Odoms-Young said that data from medical education has shown that a diverse class raises the bar for the entire class.

Mehta noted the need for a minimum set of measurable criteria to assess progress in the field on DEI issues. However, being overly prescriptive about how to address DEI and belonging will not be the most effective route because people come from different backgrounds and have different skill sets. Odoms-Young said that the only way to standardize DEI and belonging efforts is to make funding structures inclusive, for which metrics already exist.

When asked what needs to happen for children in elementary through high school to ensure they are qualified when they apply to college, Mehta said that it will be necessary to overcome the social structures and lack of resources that often disadvantage underrepresented and marginalized populations. Community engagement can help, but again, it will take intentionality to address this problem seriously and dedicate the necessary resources. Becca Jablonski said that a seed grant she received included a requirement to have the training program reviewed by a science team at the university. "I think more funders should really consider doing that, because so often the evaluation is on the outcomes of the research, which is core, but so is this training component," she said. Odoms-Young found that idea extremely interesting. "What if that was part of all awards, that you have to have some study of how are you contributing overall to the field, to knowledge, to building the field, or building teams versus just looking at research outcomes?" she wondered.

Carmen Tekwe, session moderator and associate professor of biostatistics at Indiana University at Bloomington, said that she has her students develop a statistical method and apply it to different subgroups to see if it works equally well. So far, it does not, but being exposed to the idea that statistical methods do not always apply to all populations introduces the concept of equity in research. She then has her students try to develop group-specific methods. "Many of my students would not normally be exposed to this concept of health disparities in research, but that actually gives them the ability to think about the work and how they can incorporate health disparities into the work they do," said Tekwe, who asked Mehta if there was a way to apply this approach in his training grant.

Absolutely, said Mehta. "I think that is in the spirit of the whole precision nutrition effort and trying to understand not only the different biological variability but also the variability that is accounted by the kind of methods we use." It could fit in the capstone course.

Tekwe asked how the field would know it has become more inclusive. Mehta said that it is necessary to make sure every individual feels they can thrive in this area and be comfortable with their skill set. As far as how to assess that, he said that there is no easy answer.

In closing, Rodolphe Barrangou noted the long way to go for the field in terms of DEI but there are reasons to be hopeful and ambitious. "I know there are some challenges and I know there is a long way to go for sure, but disruptive technologies like AI are going to enable us to disrupt the world at a faster pace maybe than we have been able to disrupt it until now," he said. "But I think with the right leadership, the right mentorship, the right training, the right attitude, and the right teams, we are going to get there."

5

Potential Applications of AI to Large-Scale Food and Nutrition Initiatives

> **Highlights from the Presentations of Individual Speakers**[a]
> - A concern exists about the little to no data supporting how AI-powered clinical decision tools are being used by clinicians and, for example, whether these are being used as clinical decision-making tools versus their intended use as support tools. (Hartshorn)
> - The transformational aspect of AI and ML tools will be that they change the biomedical research calculus from simply analyzing a data type and hypothesis testing to generating hypotheses from the totality of the available medical evidence. (Hartshorn)
> - The sample size for training AI systems is a long-recognized pitfall given that clinical trials typically do not recruit to the requisite sample size or demographic depth for appropriately training AI systems. (Hartshorn)
> - Agricultural producers are facing unprecedented complexity in decision making, and agricultural AI can support, but not necessarily simplify, many of those decisions. (Hipp)
> - Pitfalls and challenges associated with a failure to consider ethics, access, legal frameworks, and fairness in AI include the difficulty of recognizing and quantifying the harm caused,

> the rise of state-level pushback on AI that will lead to a patchwork of policy and an uneven policy landscape; and determining who has the right to clean up the data and how to deal with bad data and bad actors. (Hipp)
>
> ---
>
> [a] This list is the rapporteurs' summary of points made by the individual speakers identified, and the statements have not been endorsed or verified by the National Academies of Sciences, Engineering, and Medicine. They are not intended to reflect a consensus among workshop participants.

ADVANCING AI AND ML IN BIOMEDICAL RESEARCH AND HEALTH CARE AT NIH

Chris Hartshorn, chief of the digital and mobile technologies section in the National Institutes of Health (NIH) Clinical and Translational Science Awards program, discussed some challenges regarding artificial intelligence (AI) and machine learning (ML) for biomedical applications. He noted that biomedical research using ML or deep learning (DL) has accelerated rapidly over the last decade based on the literature and the number of investigator-initiated research proposals NIH has received. Another important trend is the growth, particularly over the last 7 years, in regulatory filings and U.S. Food and Drug Administration (FDA) approvals as a sign of AI and ML methods transitioning to the clinic. As of July 2023, FDA has approved nearly 700 AI/ML tools, with radiology applications accounting for 75 percent of the approvals. Hartshorn said that AI/ML tools have leapfrogged other new technologies in their path to clinical use.

Hartshorn raised the question of why dedicated public funds are still needed to support AI/ML application development, considering the accelerating translation to the clinic. One answer, he said, is that only a small percentage of the approvals used prospective data to support their request for approval (Wu et al., 2021a). Out of 130 approved AI/ML applications that one investigator examined, only 37 leveraged data from more than one site, and only four used prospective data. None of the four were for devices considered high risk. These findings, said Hartshorn, highlight some of the obvious problems with regulating these tools and the work needed to drive them to clinical utility and having measurable positive effects on clinical outcomes. Furthermore, this problem can be addressed via new approaches to clinical trials and the data produced being more AI ready or intended for an AI system and designing the trial accordingly.

Considering what is known about challenges in leveraging AI/ML for biomedical data, the data supporting approvals can be biased or incomplete, reducing the utility and accuracy of the clinical decision support (CDS) from AI/ML algorithms, which can have severe consequences if clinicians use them incorrectly, said Hartshorn. This raises other concerns about the little to no data on clinicians' usage; for example, are they ever being used for clinical *decision-making* versus the intended use as *support* tools?

Hartshorn posited several other aspects as to why this field would continue to necessitate a large body of research. The uses of AI are not focused on health across the life span as a continuous and stochastic process, and most research is narrowly focused on optimizing flow and increasing accuracy of clinical decisions for single data types, such as most approved CDS tools for radiology. Thus, the impact has largely been confined to hypothesis confirming rather than hypothesis generating, which, from his perspective, is where AI/ML will ultimately be transformative for medicine and health care writ large. "Where I think where it will be truly transformative will be its use in multimodal, disparate, big data analysis, and dot-connecting, as these are tasks, simply put, [that] humans cannot do nearly as well or at all," said Hartshorn.

The transformational aspect of AI and ML tools, he said, will be that they shift the biomedical research calculus from simply analyzing a data type and hypothesis testing to generating hypotheses from the evidence. "The ability to capture insight from the totality of medical evidence available at the individual to population level will entirely change how we deliver health care and ask research questions, yet this is by far the most challenging task, presenting a host of additional challenges to it ever being realized," said Hartshorn.

One challenge is that biomedical data are multiscale, with both spatial and temporal dimensionality, Hartshorn noted. Linking these scales is not trivial, considering that for every data scale model and link, it would be necessary to understand, mechanistically, why an AI/ML algorithm is providing a particular answer for it to have any value. Moreover, each scale has unique temporal qualities, including its inherently stochastic biological nature and also an individual's own life decisions, the decisions of others, and the environment in which they live—these present challenges to generating plausible correlations using AI/ML. As a result, all the ML and AI methods can point to correlations, but other multiscale modeling and *in vivo* experiments must be used to identify causality of correlations made by any AI system.

Hartshorn said that the second challenge is that within each scale, the data are multimodal and the tools for any individual measurement are typically not the same or even from the same vendor. In theory, AI systems have been used to generate correlations and predictions for integrated multimodal datasets before, but mostly in complex nonbiological systems. However, much remains to be done to help accelerate this for complex biological systems, said Hartshorn.

Further challenging the utility of AI in biomedical and clinical research using big data is that applying AI to biological questions requires models that can handle longitudinal, noisy, and incomplete data and a host of other aspects that are important to consider. For example, the provenance and standardization of measurements used to acquire patient data; privacy issues; categorical, nominal, and ordinal data; qualitative discrete and continuous data; and structured, semistructured, and unstructured data. Until recently, most biomedical data have not been generated with AI in mind, so little prospective data can be leveraged retrospectively. In addition, the sample size for training AI systems is a long-recognized pitfall, given that clinical trials typically do not recruit to the requisite sample size or demographic depth. How to mitigate sample size bias, such as "synthetic" data generation/injection, is still a nascent area.

Hartshorn said that with all the challenges that remain to push AI/ML to be a transformational tool in medicine, NIH is actively creating programs and funding to incentivize developing AI/ML approaches with more realistic, real-world utility in order to drive the evidence base and provide the answers to some of the challenges he noted. For at least 7 years, NIH has had many initiatives, large and small, focusing on AI/ML for biomedical research and medicine. These include the Common Fund's Nutrition for Precision Health (NPH) program, Bridge to Artificial Intelligence (Bridge2AI) program, Office of Data Science Strategy's (ODSS's) Artificial Intelligence/Machine Learning Consortium to Advance Health Equity and Researcher Diversity (AIM-AHEAD) program, and National Cancer Institute (NCI) and Department of Energy collaborations on multiple AI/ML-based programs. Bridge2AI, for example, aims to set the stage for widespread adoption of AI and tackle complex biomedical challenges by generating flagship datasets, preparing a road map for "AI/ML-friendly" data, emphasizing ethical best practices in the use of AI/ML, and promoting forming and training diverse teams. This program is developing automated tools, standardizing data elements, creating cross-training materials for workforce development, and disseminating products and best practices. Data generation projects cover topical areas, such as precision public health, functional genomics, salutogenesis, and critical care informatics. Furthermore, a myriad of smaller AI/ML programs have been established along with an ever-expanding number of successful investigator-initiated applications to NIH institutes and centers.

After briefly describing the NPH program, he mentioned that AIM-AHEAD[1] will establish mutually beneficial and coordinated partnerships to increase the participation and representation of researchers and communities underrepresented in developing AI/ML models and enhance

---

[1] Available at https://datascience.nih.gov/artificial-intelligence/aim-ahead (accessed January 9, 2024).

the capabilities of this emerging technology, beginning with electronic health record (EHR) data. Hartshorn encouraged people to go to the NIH ODSS website[2] for a continual feed of NIH's active AI-specific and related funding opportunities. He also highlighted NIH's decade-long collaboration with the National Science Foundation and Smart and Connected Health Program, which funds health-related aspects of AI and other synergistic areas in digital health.

THE NIH NPH PROGRAM

Holly Nicastro said that the goal of NPH is to develop algorithms to predict individual responses to foods and dietary patterns using data collected from 10,000 participants from diverse backgrounds on their physiology, metabolome, microbiome, genome, dietary intake, demographics, health history, psychosocial factors, behaviors, and environment. The idea is to use AI to identify the factors that explain why individuals or subgroups respond the way they do to certain foods or ways of eating. The study has an observational component that will generate data on the foods people eat in their everyday lives and an interventional component that will randomly assign participants to three dietary patterns, in their normal environments or a domiciled setting. Nicastro noted that NPH has participant ambassadors that inform the things that they would like to see studied and what they want to learn about their health.

As part of the *All of Us* Research Program, NPH will have access to its data and be able to study the techniques that Edward Sazonov, Rob Knight, and Susan McRitchie described and merge various data sources. For example, aligning the timing of food intake with metabolite changes may provide information on how the metabolome changes over time.

Privacy and trust are concerns, said Nicastro, given that some studies will ask participants to wear cameras that may capture other people. "We also need to be aware of the increasing possibility of identifiability with the data we are collecting," she said. "We are building more and more toward having digital twins or digital avatars of ourselves, so we are starting to blur the boundaries of what could be considered personal identifiable information." In addition, as this work may provide information on disease risk, it will be important to remember that this does not equal disease and exercise caution about any potential stigma or insurance-related issues.

Nicastro said that the program does not want to identify and troubleshoot issues of privacy and trust in real time. "We want to be taking proactive approaches to build trust versus assuming that we are starting with that trust and then losing it," she said. Regarding diversity, equity,

---

[2] Available at https://datascience.nih.gov/artificial-intelligence (accessed January 9, 2024).

and inclusion (DEI) and accessibility, she sees a tremendous opportunity for advances in data collection to engage people who have not participated in nutrition studies before and ensure that any findings are relevant to and reach diverse populations. "We all need to be considering how any of these big data findings can be translated and implemented in clinic and community settings and not just for those with disposable income," she said. One possibility is developing simple point-of-care technologies, perhaps a finger prick, that can capture a simple metabolomic signature to better inform personalized nutrition recommendations.

Nicastro is also excited about the ability of passive image-assisted technologies to provide a fuller picture of what participants are eating to complement self-reported behavior. As technologies such as smart toilets or smarter fecal sample collection devices improve, they may address barriers, such as people's reluctance to collect fecal samples or store their biospecimens in the refrigerator before their clinic visit.

Collaborations will be critical to moving the field forward, said Nicastro. "We need nutrition scientists in the same room with the engineers, but beyond bringing people together, we need cross-training of the workforce," she said. Regarding where the field might be in 5–10 years, she wondered if it is overpromising or being realistic. "Are we going to walk into a restaurant, pull out our phone, access our digital twin, and maybe simulate what will happen to our cardiovascular risk profile if we order the burger versus the salad? Probably not," said Nicastro. But she is certain that initial results from NPH will power algorithms that provide a better understanding of why some people respond in certain ways to food.

The immediate next steps, said Nicastro, will be to validate algorithms in different populations and settings and conduct trials to see if targeted guidance based on these algorithms produce the desired results. That could lead to including predictors and the evidence behind them in the *Dietary Guidelines for Americans*, which would be a great example of precision nutrition. The idea, she added, is for practitioners to use this information to inform dietary advice, whether that is the calorie level an individual might need or the foods they should eat.

Tempering her excitement about the future of precision nutrition are the realities of health care delivery today, where physicians are spending less time with patients while being asked to explain ever more complicated topics, such as computer-generated risk profiles. "When we start to add in more of these personalization or precision factors for a patient, is this going to be more burdensome for the practitioner and the patient, or will knowing that this advice was tailored to that individual serve as a tool to make them better empowered to stick to their plan?" asked Nicastro. "We will find out."

ETHICS, ACCESS, LEGAL FRAMEWORKS, AND FAIRNESS IN AI

Janie Hipp, inaugural president and chief executive officer of Native Agriculture Financial Services, began by noting that agricultural producers are facing unprecedented complexity in decision making and that agricultural AI could support, but not necessarily simplify, many of those decisions (Sørensen et al., 2010). Agricultural production, she added, is a data- and algorithm-intensive process, and AI encounters every challenge that speakers have discussed about dealing with big data systems (Ayoub Shaikh et al., 2022). Analyzing and absorbing the copious amounts of data into farm production systems will be essential to achieve a fair, just, and efficient system of food production in the United States. "We cannot get this wrong, or we are headed for a picture of a very unfair, unjust food system writ large," she said.

Hipp explained that approximately 6 percent of agricultural producers account for 60–70 percent of the nation's agricultural output. The other 94 percent fall in the small to mid-size category[3] but have the same challenges as large-scale producers. However, the needs of the farm manager and ranch manager will be different based on the size and nature of their operations.

The architecture of smart agriculture is complex, and farmer decisions are driven by environmental, market, and cultural conditions and any available data (see Figure 5-1). The farm household, said Hipp, is where human health and decisions around food, food preparation, consumption, and nutrition collide with what is happening on the farm as a component of the farm system. "That is a very interesting place to be, because how you believe farmers actually respond to data can be quite different in real life than what you think it is going to be as you are researching this arena and trying to contemplate their reactions," said Hipp.

Hipp listed several questions regarding the role of government regulation and safeguards:

- Who owns the data that will drive these innovations?
- Who owns the innovations derived from these data?
- Who is responsible for ensuring the veracity of the AI systems?
- Who is responsible for security of the AI systems?
- What is the legal framework that surrounds AI?
- What is the ethical framework that surrounds AI?

As Hipp noted, agriculture is inherently data rich, with farmers generating data every single day from the land, their equipment, their inputs,

---

[3] Available at https://www.ers.usda.gov/data-products/chart-gallery/gallery/chart-detail/?chartId=108013 (accessed December 29, 2023).

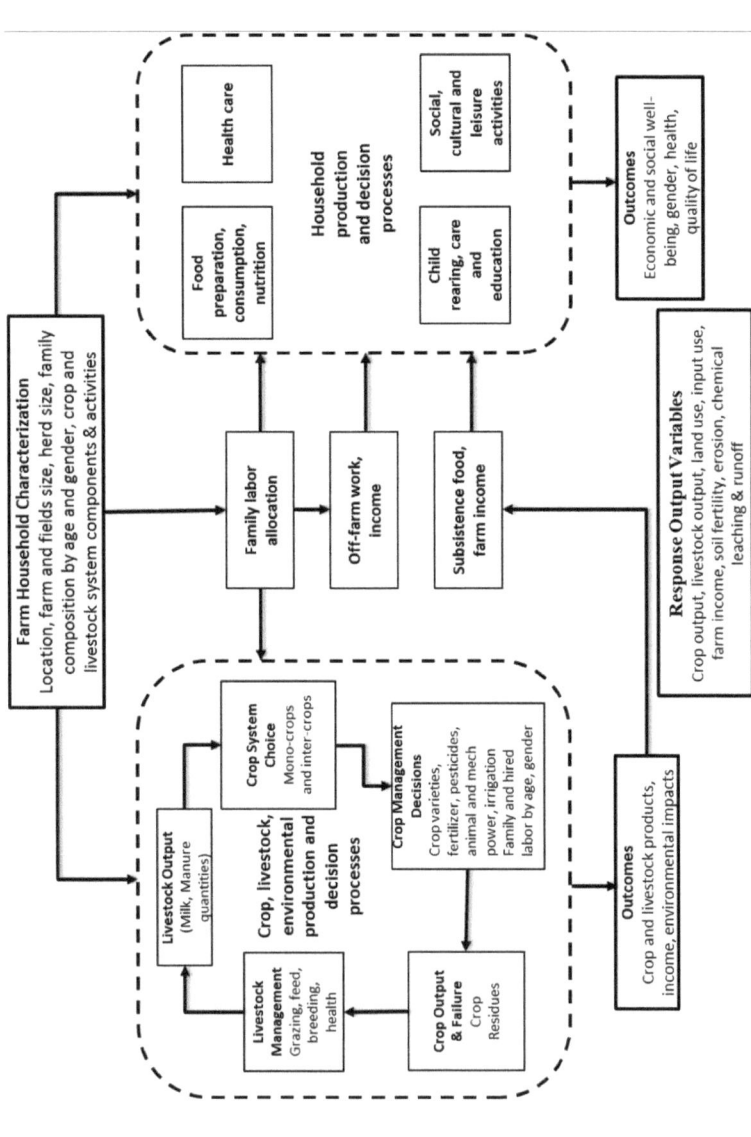

FIGURE 5-1 The complex nature of farm decisions.
SOURCE: Presented by Janie Hipp on October 11, 2024, at the workshop on The Role of Advanced Computation, Predictive Technologies, and Big Data Analytics in Food and Nutrition Research; Jones et al., 2017.

and their labor. How they do so will depend on whether they own the land and operation or just manage or work on it. Many people involved in farm production have questions about the producer's ownership rights associated with an AI model if it is built with data the producer owns. For example, who owns it, at which stage in the creation process does ownership or shared ownership attach, and where does the government come in during this process? What happens when the data used to create the AI model are bad? How do bad data affect the farmer whose raw data go into the AI?

Another important question concerns the national security implications of AI in agriculture, given that food security is national security and AI will affect food security, food access and availability, and success of the sector. For example, what aspects of data and AI in agriculture have national security implications? Those implications lead Hipp to believe that government must be involved. "We have to get this piece of the puzzle right," she said.

One problem Hipp has seen as a lawyer is that farmers and ranchers sign nonnegotiable contracts to obtain the equipment and supplies they need to continue their operations. What this means is that although 77 and 80 percent of them are worried about data security and believe they own their own data (Yu et al., 2021), respectively, they actually do not according to the contracts she has seen and analyzed. "Ownership and control of farming data is a significant concern for me, and it should be at the policy level," said Hipp. "It allows for market speculation and control of ag operations, and it can start to spin off into national security issues very quickly." It also feeds into her concern about bad data.

As an example of the harm that a farmer can experience from bad actors using their data, Hipp explained that farmers regularly participate in the agricultural census and with research communities in on-farm demonstration projects that generate data for use by other farmers and ranchers. In the 1990s and 2000s, data mining resulted in environmental lawsuits directed at farmers who had for decades poured their data into publicly accessible datasets and did things in a certain way based on feedback from the research community. Despite identity protection laws, the small set of farmers makes it fairly easy to figure out who generated the data.

Hipp explained that the legal mechanisms for dealing with how U.S. law protects data in the realm of AI do not exist. In her opinion, patent, trademark, and copyright laws are not set up to deal with the reality of AI. She explained that U.S. law classifies data as facts (Yu et al., 2021). As the basic facts underlying certain agricultural commodities, farm data lack a creative element that can be defined as an intellectual property whose ownership could be protected by copyright laws. Therefore, legally speaking, farmers may not own their raw data. Hipp noted that patent, trademark, and copyright laws are controlled at the federal level, and trade secret issues are primarily controlled by state laws.

States have passed laws to protect data at the farm gate level so they could not be used by outside forces against the farmer or rancher in a way that affects what they do. What concerns Hipp is a possible patchwork of state laws that will cause an uneven growth trajectory for AI.

Hipp said that the driving force for her work and involvement has been that agricultural production improvement has always been about stemming the tide of hunger and malnutrition, although agriculture is not just an economic act but an act of community, sacredness, and protection of one another. However, it can be a means of exploiting communities and people. That raises the issue of the interaction with and impact on the AI model of the most underserved actors. Hipp said that it is hard to consider ethics in AI without confronting the nebulous concepts of community, sacredness, and protection. "I fear for us if we do not insist that these unseen forces for why people make the decisions that they do are a part of the conversation," she said.

The other piece of this puzzle that troubles Hipp is that data and AI/ML applications are only usable if one has the time and space, and the larger players are more able to actually absorb data and applications into their operations and make decisions with that data. "But if you are at a smaller end of an agricultural operation, you are many times operating on knowing your gut and what is happening right at that moment. You do not have the luxury or the time or the money, literally, to ponder the data," said Hipp. This issue raises questions:

- How to target AI both at the larger players and simultaneously at the vast numbers of smaller players?
- How to stabilize access to data and information?
- How to ensure AI is size specific?
- Is the goal to improve the lives of the entire community or only a limited set of people?

Hipp added that if it is too hard to consider ethics in AI, the nation must be prepared to live with the outcomes.

Legal frameworks, said Hipp, must be reformed at the same time society embraces its AI future in agriculture. Questions that need answering include the following:

- What is the regulatory regime, and who holds it?
- How to ensure privacy of data generated on the farm?
- How to ensure permissions/authorizations for using data occur, and if compensation for data is provided, how do we ensure the amount is fair?

- How to focus on incentives in AI and not just regulation? Are incentives the only approach that allows for the continued presence of small to mid-sized players?
- What are the unintended consequences to various types/sizes of producers as AI proceeds?
- How to ensure informed consent for using data?
- A solely "regulatory" approach to the output of AI will further ensure uneven distribution of AI. How do we safeguard against this?
- AI can affect environmental management, risk management, economic analysis, resiliency, and adaptation to climate change; which of these have the greatest potential for harm and need the greater level of regulation and scrutiny?

Hipp said that in her opinion, the U.S. Department of Agriculture (USDA) is the only informed choice regarding regulation of AI and agriculture. However, USDA does not oversee regulatory regimes and deals more with incentives rather than regulations.

Not considering ethics, access, legal frameworks, and fairness in AI will lead to exploitation, said Hipp, and prevent accessing inherent knowing and sacredness, which is a huge issue for Indigenous communities such as hers. "There is a deep, deep understanding within Indigenous communities and tribal governments in the United States that data sovereignty is important, and we are very highly concerned about these issues," she said. The conversation about data ownership and AI is just starting in the native producer community.

Other pitfalls and challenges associated with a failure to consider ethics, access, legal frameworks, and fairness in AI include the difficulty of recognizing and quantifying the harm caused; the rise of state-level pushback that will lead to a patchwork of policy and an uneven policy landscape; determining who has the right to clean up the data and how to deal with bad data and bad actors; and the question of who is at the table throughout the discussions to embed fairness in AI policies and who is creating the decision support systems that allow producers to stop drowning in their data and start using them. Datasets in agriculture production are almost unusable by the farmers who generate the data and can experience the most improvement in the resiliency and viability of their operations, said Hipp.

Hipp pointed to the need to attend to the DEI, accessibility, and fairness of AI systems as they are being built, modified, and enlarged. Competent lawyers are needed at the table now, as is impressing upon lawmakers at every level that this train is moving fast and, without a focus on achieving the proper balance today, agriculture is headed for a rapid exacerbation of exclusion, exploitation, lack of privacy, and failures of control. Finally, she said, "If we have any hope of a fair and just food system that takes into account national and food security and that achieves the highest good for the most people, we must get this right."

MODERATED DISCUSSION

When asked if he sees any pitfalls regarding the program NIH is funding on the use of AI in nutrition (NPH program), Hartshorn said that he does not, given this is discovery-based versus strictly hypothesis-driven science—unique to traditional NIH efforts. Hipp largely agreed with Hartshorn but also wondered if advances in biomedicine and nutrition will send market signals back into the food system writ large and change what farmers grow, how and where they grow it, and even who grows it. The challenge, she said, is making any transitions as fluid and least harmful as possible and providing incentives that allow farmers and ranchers to be full participants in the AI arena in a way that does not exacerbate concentration in agriculture.

Hipp said that her vision for the future is to have a tool that a farmer standing in a field and wondering how to deal with a certain circumstance can use to get various options that will guide them in a way that does not harm their operation. In addition, all producers, regardless of their size, will have access to the same set of decision support tools. That would allow small and mid-size producers to have a viable path forward and stay on the land and continue producing food. She added that as an Indigenous person, it is important that whatever gets developed, it must acknowledge that she is different, that each person is an individual.

6

Final Discussion and Synthesis

Sharon Kirkpatrick began with a review of the workshop's goals, which were to discuss promising opportunities and directions and best-known practices in the application of advanced computation, big data analytics, and high-performance computing to food and nutrition research; consider likely pitfalls, including those associated with privacy, bias, and trust, and safeguards to avoid them; reflect on the appropriate use of evidence generated by these methods; and consider needed investments in capacity development. She summarized some of the workshop's main themes:

- Applying artificial intelligence (AI), machine learning (ML), and deep learning (DL) to food and nutrition research is a series of interrelated moonshots, with both optimism and pessimism that these moonshots will succeed
- Making existing data more available, improving the representation of ongoing data collection, and addressing issues of data sovereignty
- Assembling diverse teams that collaborate and communicate effectively and develop a shared vocabulary and culture
- Engaging communities and other stakeholders early in study design
- Developing and using AI/ML/DL tools in a manner that supports equity, fairness, and justice for all end users and reflects the broader context of social and structural determinants of health and nutrition
- AI is useful, but it is not magic and requires human expertise to be most useful

Christopher Mejía-Argueta agreed with Kirkpatrick's summary and emphasized the importance of ensuring that technology, data, and model-driven strategies include input from stakeholder communities and will benefit the smallholder farmers, retailers, and family-owned businesses, which will have a role in including nutrition in the food ecosystem. Sai Krupa Das noted that the research community has developed useful AI-enabled tools and is smart enough to recognize that data are messy and have gaps and to work together to fix this. With those tools, the field can develop the infrastructure that will enable moving toward the end goal of improving human health while benefiting the planet. She recognized the possible legal and ethical pitfalls that Janie Hipp discussed and the importance of ensuring that data and models are not exploited in ways that harm agricultural producers by making a concerted effort regarding data surveillance, data monitoring, stewardship, and equitable access.

Angela Odoms-Young wondered how AI could help shape food assistance and production policies so they reflect the differential responses that various subpopulations have to food intake and nutritional advice. By focusing on subpopulations rather than individuals, such policies may transform the structures that contribute to inequity.

Rodolphe Barrangou reiterated that foundational AI tools exist and, although they can be adapted and improved, they have established a sound platform and basis for use. The main limitations in his view concern the data. Yes, data are abundant, but they are not always accessible, formatted properly, of the highest quality, curated, or regulated correctly. He also expressed concern about how those working in the field in different disciplines can better collaborate and develop a common language and culture and said that the field needs to involve nutritionists, clinicians, data analysts, food scientists, farmers and ranchers, public relations experts, social scientists, behavioral scientists, economists, supply chain experts, and marketing and communications experts. He called for incentivizing people from these disciplines to join the teams needed to harness nutrition and food to preventively manage health as opposed to curing disease. "I think we need to strategize about the who and the how we are going to work together to be more efficient," said Barrangou.

Kirkpatrick noted the general lack of institutional support for team-based science and wondered how to address this problem. Mejía-Argueta acknowledged that this is a difficult situation and suggested ways to bolster team performance:

- Identifying the key performance indicators for each member and similarities across the team that can be leveraged to benefit everyone regarding institutional recognition, perhaps by enabling different members to serve as the primary author on publications reporting the findings.

- Using grant funds to collaborate with colleagues from countries outside of the United States that face similar problems and challenges.
- Inviting people from industry or nonprofit organizations to provide feedback on programmatic activities to expose team members to the need to ensure that the team's work needs to be useful.
- Gaining the trust of others to create alliances that are sustainable over the long term and can create their own key performance indicators.
- Developing a culture that creates synergies and ensures the team is robust and able to address the same problem from different perspectives.

Das noted that everyone may not be equipped or would need to start assembling large teams but could be ready to contribute to efforts that would benefit from their domain expertise and that this will require keeping up with and understanding the landscape and comprehensive nature of ongoing research and providing expertise within that context. Odoms-Young noted the movement at some institutions to change the key performance indicators used for promotion and tenure decisions to reflect the value of team-based research or community-based participatory research, for example. The key is having the right metrics of success in place, which perhaps professional organizations could develop to reflect new ways of engaging in research.

Barrangou agreed about changes to promotion and tenure metrics and called for the community to build new infrastructures to support this growing field. Odoms-Young added that policy makers have also begun to change how they decide on where grant funds go, but the field needs to do more to engage them and the public to show the value that team science creates. Das said that the tide is changing in a way that empowers trainees and early career investigators to push for new infrastructures and new norms regarding promotion and tenure.

Aaron Smith said that deep disciplinary expertise is needed for the field to realize its potential. Therefore, Smith continued, it is important to ensure that training does not dilute that by only producing people who are good at everything; generalists help disciplinary experts talk to one another.

References

Alexander, C. S., A. Smith, and R. Ivanek. 2023a. Safer not to know?: Shaping liability law and policy to incentivize adoption of predictive AI technologies in the food system. *Frontiers in Artificial Intelligence* 6:1298604.

Alexander, C., M. Yarborough, and A. Smith. 2023b. Who is responsible for "responsible AI"?: Navigating challenges to build trust in AI agriculture and food system technology. *Precision Agriculture* 1–40.

Ayoub Shaikh, T., T. Rasool, and F. Rasheed Lone. 2022. Towards leveraging the role of machine learning and artificial intelligence in precision agriculture and smart farming. *Computers and Electronics in Agriculture* 198:107119.

Azarianpour Esfahani, S., P. Fu, H. Mahdi, and A. Madabhushi. 2021. Computational features of TIL architecture are differentially prognostic of uterine cancer between African and Caucasian American women. *Journal of Clinical Oncology* 39(15_suppl):5585.

Bathgate, K. E., J. L. Sherriff, H. Leonard, S. S. Dhaliwal, E. J. Delp, C. J. Boushey, and D. A. Kerr. 2017. Feasibility of assessing diet with a mobile food record for adolescents and young adults with Down Syndrome. *Nutrients* 9(3).

Ben-Yacov, O., A. Godneva, M. Rein, S. Shilo, D. Kolobkov, N. Koren, N. Cohen Dolev, T. Travinsky Shmul, B. C. Wolf, N. Kosower, K. Sagiv, M. Lotan-Pompan, N. Zmora, A. Weinberger, E. Elinav, and E. Segal. 2021. Personalized postprandial glucose response-targeting diet versus Mediterranean diet for glycemic control in prediabetes. *Diabetes Care* 44(9):1980–1991.

Bera, K., N. Braman, A. Gupta, V. Velcheti, and A. Madabhushi. 2022. Predicting cancer outcomes with radiomics and artificial intelligence in radiology. *Nature Reviews: Clinical Oncology* 19(2):132–146.

Brown, A. G. M., S. Shi, S. Adas, J. E. A. Boyington, P. A. Cotton, B. Jirles, N. Rajapakse, J. Reedy, K. Regan, D. Xi, G. Zappalà, and T. Agurs-Collins. 2022. A decade of nutrition and health disparities research at NIH, 2010–2019. *American Journal of Preventive Medicine* 63(2):e49–e57.

Cech, E. A., and T. J. Waidzunas. 2021. Systemic inequalities for LGBTQ professionals in STEM. *Science Advances* 7(3):eabe0933. https://doi.org/10.1126/sciadv.abe0933.

Chen, G., W. Jia, Y. Zhao, Z. H. Mao, B. Lo, A. K. Anderson, G. Frost, M. L. Jobarteh, M. A. McCrory, E. Sazonov, M. Steiner-Asiedu, R. S. Ansong, T. Baranowski, L. Burke, and M. Sun. 2021. Food/non-food classification of real-life egocentric images in low- and middle-income countries based on image tagging features. *Frontiers in Artificial X_Inteligence* 4:644712.

Coleman-Jensen, A., M. Rabbitt, C. Gregory, and A. Singh. 2022. *Household food security in the United States in 2021*. ERR-309. U.S. Department of Agriculture, Economic Research Service. https://www.ers.usda.gov/publications/pub-details/?pubid=104655 (accessed December 26, 2023).

Côté, M., and B. Lamarche. 2021. Artificial intelligence in nutrition research: Perspectives on current and future applications. *Applied Physiology, Nutrition, and Metabolism* 1–8.

Côté, M., M. A. Osseni, D. Brassard, É. Carbonneau, J. Robitaille, M. C. Vohl, S. Lemieux, F. Laviolette, and B. Lamarche. 2022. Are machine learning algorithms more accurate in predicting vegetable and fruit consumption than traditional statistical models? An exploratory analysis. *Frontiers in Nutrition* 9:740898.

Das, S. 2021. *Delivering locally sourced nutritious food to Indian households*. MIT. https://ctl.mit.edu/pub/thesis/delivering-locally-sourced-nutritious-food-indian-households (accessed December 26, 2023).

de la Cuesta-Zuluaga, J., S. T. Kelley, Y. Chen, J. S. Escobar, N. T. Mueller, R. E. Ley, D. McDonald, S. Huang, A. D. Swafford, R. Knight, and V. G. Thackray. 2019. Age- and sex-dependent patterns of gut microbial diversity in human adults. *mSystems* 4(4).

DeGrave, A. J., J. D. Janizek, and S.-I. Lee. 2021. AI for radiographic COVID-19 detection selects shortcuts over signal. *Nature Machine Intelligence* 3(7):610–619.

Dhamdhere, R., G. Modanwal, M. H. E. Makhlouf, N. S. Hassani, S. Bharadwaj, P. Fu, I. Milloglou, M. Rahman, S. Al-Kindi, and A. Madabhushi. 2023. *STAR-echo: A novel biomarker for prognosis of MACE in chronic kidney disease patients using spatiotemporal analysis and transformer-based radiomics models*. Paper presented at Medical Image Computing and Computer-Assisted Intervention 2023: 26th International Conference, Vancouver, BC.

Dong, V., D. D. Sevgi, S. S. Kar, S. K. Srivastava, J. P. Ehlers, and A. Madabhushi. 2022. Evaluating the utility of deep learning for predicting therapeutic response in diabetic eye disease. *Frontiers in Ophthalmology* 2:852107. https://doi.org/10.3389/fopht.2022.852107.

Dong, Y., A. Hoover, J. Scisco, and E. Muth. 2012. A new method for measuring meal intake in humans via automated wrist motion tracking. *Applied Psychophysiology and Biofeedback* 37(3):205–215.

Doulah, A., M. Farooq, X. Yang, J. Parton, M. A. McCrory, J. A. Higgins, and E. Sazonov. 2017. Meal microstructure characterization from sensor-based food intake detection. *Frontiers in Nutrition* 4:31.

Doulah, A., T. Ghosh, D. Hossain, M. Imtiaz, and E. Sazonov. 2021. "Automatic ingestion monitor version 2"—a novel wearable device for automatic food intake detection and passive capture of food images. *IEEE Journal of Biomedical and Health Informatics* 25(2):568–576.

Doulah, A., T. Ghosh, D. Hossain, T. Marden, J. M. Parton, J. A. Higgins, M. A. McCrory, and E. Sazonov. 2022. Energy intake estimation using a novel wearable sensor and food images in a laboratory (pseudo-free-living) meal setting: Quantification and contribution of sources of error. *International Journal of Obesity* 46(11):2050–2057.

Dratsch, T., X. Chen, M. R. Mehrizi, R. Kloeckner, A. Mähringer-Kunz, M. Püsken, B. Baeßler, S. Sauer, D. Maintz, and D. Pinto dos Santos. 2023. Automation bias in mammography: The impact of artificial intelligence BI-RADS suggestions on reader performance. *Radiology* 307(4):e222176.

Drukker, K., W. Chen, J. Gichoya, N. Gruszauskas, J. Kalpathy-Cramer, S. Koyejo, K. Myers, R. C. Sá, B. Sahiner, H. Whitney, Z. Zhang, and M. Giger. 2023. Toward fairness in artificial intelligence for medical image analysis: Identification and mitigation of potential biases in the roadmap from data collection to model deployment. *Journal of Medical Imaging* 10(6):061104.

FAO (Food and Agriculture Organization). 2020. *The state of food security and nutrition in the world 2020. Transforming food systems for affordable healthy diets.* Rome: FAO. https://doi.org/10.4060/ca9692en (accessed January 9, 2024).

Farooq, M., and E. Sazonov. 2017. Segmentation and characterization of chewing bouts by monitoring temporalis muscle using smart glasses with piezoelectric sensor. *IEEE Journal of Biomedical Health Information* 21(6):1495–1503.

Farooq, M., J. M. Fontana, and E. Sazonov. 2014. A novel approach for food intake detection using electroglottography. *Physiological Measurement* 35(5):739–751.

Farooq, M., P. C. Chandler-Laney, M. Hernandez-Reif, and E. Sazonov. 2015. Monitoring of infant feeding behavior using a jaw motion sensor. *Journal of Healthcare Engineering* 6(1):23–40.

Garaulet, M., P. Gómez-Abellán, J. J. Alburquerque-Béjar, Y. C. Lee, J. M. Ordovás, and F. A. Scheer. 2013. Timing of food intake predicts weight loss effectiveness. *International Journal of Obesity* 37(4):604–611.

Garaulet, M., B. Vera, G. Bonnet-Rubio, P. Gomez-Abellan, Y. C. Lee, and J. M. Ordovas. 2016. Lunch eating predicts weight-loss effectiveness in carriers of the common allele at PERILIPIN1: The ONTIME (Obesity, Nutrigenetics, Timing, Mediterranean) study. *American Journal of Clinical Nutrition* 104(4):1160–1166.

Gauglitz, J. M., K. A. West, W. Bittremieux, C. L. Williams, K. C. Weldon, M. Panitchpakdi, F. Di Ottavio, C. M. Aceves, E. Brown, N. C. Sikora, A. K. Jarmusch, C. Martino, A. Tripathi, M. J. Meehan, K. Dorrestein, J. P. Shaffer, R. Coras, F. Vargas, L. D. Goldasich, T. Schwartz, M. Bryant, G. Humphrey, A. J. Johnson, K. Spengler, P. Belda-Ferre, E. Diaz, D. McDonald, Q. Zhu, E. O. Elijah, M. Wang, C. Marotz, K. E. Sprecher, D. Vargas-Robles, D. Withrow, G. Ackermann, L. Herrera, B. J. Bradford, L. M. M. Marques, J. G. Amaral, R. M. Silva, F. P. Veras, T. M. Cunha, R. D. R. Oliveira, P. Louzada-Junior, R. H. Mills, P. K. Piotrowski, S. L. Servetas, S. M. Da Silva, C. M. Jones, N. J. Lin, K. A. Lippa, S. A. Jackson, R. K. Daouk, D. Galasko, P. S. Dulai, T. I. Kalashnikova, C. Wittenberg, R. Terkeltaub, M. M. Doty, J. H. Kim, K. E. Rhee, J. Beauchamp-Walters, K. P. Wright, M. G. Dominguez-Bello, M. Manary, M. F. Oliveira, B. S. Boland, N. P. Lopes, M. Guma, A. D. Swafford, R. J. Dutton, R. Knight, and P. C. Dorrestein. 2022. Enhancing untargeted metabolomics using metadata-based source annotation. *Nature Biotechnology* 40(12):1774–1779.

Gelaye, B., S. J. Sumner, S. McRitchie, J. E. Carlson, C. V. Ananth, D. A. Enquobahrie, C. Qiu, T. K. Sorensen, and M. A. Williams. 2016. Maternal early pregnancy serum metabolomics profile and abnormal vaginal bleeding as predictors of placental abruption: A prospective study. *PloS One* 11(6):e0156755.

Ghanbari, R., Y. Li, W. Pathmasiri, S. McRitchie, A. Etemadi, J. D. Pollock, H. Poustchi, A. Rahimi-Movaghar, M. Amin-Esmaeili, G. Roshandel, A. Shayanrad, B. Abaei, R. Malekzadeh, and S. C. J. Sumner. 2021. Metabolomics reveals biomarkers of opioid use disorder. *Translational Psychiatry* 11(1):103.

Ghosh, T., D. Hossain, and E. Sazonov. 2021. Detection of food intake sensor's wear compliance in free-living. *IEEE Sensors Journal* 21(24):27728–27735.

Gichoya, J. W., I. Banerjee, A. R. Bhimireddy, J. L. Burns, L. A. Celi, L. C. Chen, R. Correa, N. Dullerud, M. Ghassemi, S. C. Huang, P. C. Kuo, M. P. Lungren, L. J. Palmer, B. J. Price, S. Purkayastha, A. T. Pyrros, L. Oakden-Rayner, C. Okechukwu, L. Seyyed-Kalantari, H. Trivedi, R. Wang, Z. Zaiman, and H. Zhang. 2022. AI recognition of patient race in medical imaging: A modelling study. *Lancet Digital Health* 4(6):e406–e414.

Hassan, M. A., and E. Sazonov. 2020. Selective content removal for egocentric wearable camera in nutritional studies. *IEEE Access* 8:198615–198623.

He, Y., C. Xu, N. Khanna, C. J. Boushey, and E. J. Delp. 2013. Food image analysis: Segmentation, identification and weight estimation. *Proceedings of the IEEE International Conference on Multimedia and Expo.* https://doi.org/10.1109/ICME.2013.6607548.

Hoppe, T. A., A. Litovitz, K. A. Willis, R. A. Meseroll, M. J. Perkins, B. I. Hutchins, A. F. Davis, M. S. Lauer, H. A. Valantine, J. M. Anderson, and G. M. Santangelo. 2019. Topic choice contributes to the lower rate of NIH awards to African-American/Black scientists. *Science Advances* 5(10):eaaw7238.

Hossain, D., T. Ghosh, M. H. Imtiaz, and E. Sazonov. 2023. Ear canal pressure sensor for food intake detection. *Frontiers in Electronics* 4:1173607.

Hussar, B., J. Zhang, S. Hein, K. Wang, A. Robers, J. Cui, M. Smith, F. Bullock Mann, A. Barmer, and R. Dilig. 2020. *The condition of education 2020.* Washington, DC: National Center for Education Statistics.

Jones, J. W., J. M. Antle, B. Basso, K. J. Boote, R. T. Conant, I. Foster, H. C. J. Godfray, M. Herrero, R. E. Howitt, S. Janssen, B. A. Keating, R. Munoz-Carpena, C. H. Porter, C. Rosenzweig, and T. R. Wheeler. 2017. Toward a new generation of agricultural system data, models, and knowledge products: State of agricultural systems science. *Agricultural Systems* 155:269–288.

Kalantarian, H., N. Alshurafa, T. Le, and M. Sarrafzadeh. 2015. Monitoring eating habits using a piezoelectric sensor-based necklace. *Computers in Biology and Medicine* 58:46–55.

Kandori, A., T. Yamamoto, Y. Sano, M. Oonuma, T. Miyashita, M. Murata, and S. Sakoda. 2012. Simple magnetic swallowing detection system. *IEEE Sensors Journal* 12(4):805–811.

Kelly, P., S. J. Marshall, H. Badland, J. Kerr, M. Oliver, A. R. Doherty, and C. Foster. 2013. An ethical framework for automated, wearable cameras in health behavior research. *American Journal of Preventive Medicine* 44(3):314–319.

Kirk, D., E. Kok, M. Tufano, B. Tekinerdogan, E. J. M. Feskens, and G. Camps. 2022. Machine learning in nutrition research. *Advances in Nutrition* 13(6):2573–2589.

Knights, D., L. W. Parfrey, J. Zaneveld, C. Lozupone, and R. Knight. 2011. Human-associated microbial signatures: Examining their predictive value. *Cell Host & Microbe* 10(4):292–296.

Kumanyika, S. K., M. C. Whitt-Glover, T. L. Gary, T. E. Prewitt, A. M. Odoms-Young, J. Banks-Wallace, B. M. Beech, C. H. Halbert, N. Karanja, K. J. Lancaster, and C. D. Samuel-Hodge. 2007. Expanding the obesity research paradigm to reach African American communities. *Preventing Chronic Disease* 4(4):A112.

Lee, B. Y., J. M. Ordovás, E. J. Parks, C. A. M. Anderson, A. L. Barabási, S. K. Clinton, K. de la Haye, V. B. Duffy, P. W. Franks, E. M. Ginexi, K. J. Hammond, E. C. Hanlon, M. Hittle, E. Ho, A. L. Horn, R. S. Isaacson, P. L. Mabry, S. Malone, C. K. Martin, J. Mattei, S. N. Meydani, L. M. Nelson, M. L. Neuhouser, B. Parent, N. P. Pronk, H. M. Roche, M. Saria, F. Scheer, E. Segal, M. A. Sevick, T. D. Spector, L. Van Horn, K. A. Varady, V. S. Voruganti, and M. F. Martinez. 2022. Research gaps and opportunities in precision nutrition: An NIH workshop report. *American Journal of Clinical Nutrition* 116(6):1877–1900.

Lee, T., E. Puyol-Antón, B. Ruijsink, K. Aitcheson, M. Shi, and A. P. King. 2023. An investigation into the impact of deep learning model choice on sex and race bias in cardiac MR segmentation. In *Clinical image-based procedures, fairness of AI in medical imaging, and ethical and philosophical issues in medical imaging*, edited by S. Wesarg. Switzerland: Springer Nature. Pp. 215–224.

Li, H., K. Bera, H. Gilmore, N. E. Davidson, L. J. Goldstein, and A. Madabhushi. 2020. Abstract p5-06-16: Histomorphometric measure of disorder of collagen fiber orientation is associated with risk of recurrence in ER+ breast cancers in ECOG-ACRIN e2197 and TCGA-BRCA. *Cancer Research* 80(4_Supplement):P5-06-16.

Li, H., K. Bera, P. Toro, P. Fu, V. Rao, S. Siddique, A. Harbhajanka, H. Sechrist, Z. Zhang, S. Desai, V. Parmar, and A. Madabhushi. 2021a. Computerized image analysis of nuclear morphological features reveals differences in phenotype and prognosis of disease free survival of early stage ER+ breast cancers for South Asian and North American women. *Cancer Research* 81(4_Supplement):PS4-45.

Li, H., K. Bera, P. Toro, P. Fu, Z. Zhang, C. Lu, M. Feldman, S. Ganesan, L. J. Goldstein, N. E. Davidson, A. Glasgow, A. Harbhajanka, H. Gilmore, and A. Madabhushi. 2021b. Collagen fiber orientation disorder from H&E images is prognostic for early stage breast cancer: Clinical trial validation. *NPJ Breast Cancer* 7(1):104.

Li, Y. Y., R. Ghanbari, W. Pathmasiri, S. McRitchie, H. Poustchi, A. Shayanrad, G. Roshandel, A. Etemadi, J. D. Pollock, R. Malekzadeh, and S. C. J. Sumner. 2020. Untargeted metabolomics: Biochemical perturbations in Golestan cohort study opium users inform intervention strategies. *Frontiers in Nutrition* 7:584585.

Liu, J., E. Johns, L. Atallah, C. Pettitt, B. Lo, G. Frost, and G. Z. Yang. 2012. An intelligent food-intake monitoring system using wearable sensors. Paper read at 2012 Ninth International Conference on Wearable and Implantable Body Sensor Networks, May 9–12, 2012. London, UK.

Lo, F. P. W., Y. Sun, J. Qiu, and B. Lo. 2020. Image-based food classification and volume estimation for dietary assessment: A review. *IEEE Journal of Biomedical and Health Informatics* 24(7):1926–1939.

Loeser, R. F., L. Arbeeva, K. Kelley, A. A. Fodor, S. Sun, V. Ulici, L. Longobardi, Y. Cui, D. A. Stewart, S. J. Sumner, M. A. Azcarate-Peril, R. B. Sartor, I. M. Carroll, J. B. Renner, J. M. Jordan, and A. E. Nelson. 2022. Association of increased serum lipopolysaccharide, but not microbial dysbiosis, with obesity-related osteoarthritis. *Arthritis and Rheumatology* 74(2):227–236.

Loos, R. J. 2012. Genetic determinants of common obesity and their value in prediction. *Best Practice & Research: Clinical Endocrinology & Metabolism* 26(2):211–226.

Lorenzo, R., N. Voigt, K. Schetelig, A. Zawadzki, I. Welpe, and P. Brosi. 2017. *The mix that matters: Innovation through diversity*. Boston, MA: Boston Consulting Group.

Lu, C., H. Xu, J. Xu, H. Gilmore, M. Mandal, and A. Madabhushi. 2016. Multi-pass adaptive voting for nuclei detection in histopathological images. *Scientific Reports* 6:33985.

Makeyev, O., P. Lopez-Meyer, S. Schuckers, W. Besio, and E. Sazonov. 2012. Automatic food intake detection based on swallowing sounds. *Biomedical Signal Processing and Control* 7(6):649–656.

Marin, J., A. Biswas, F. Ofli, N. Hynes, A. Salvador, Y. Aytar, I. Weber, and A. Torralba. 2021. Recipe1M+: A dataset for learning cross-modal embeddings for cooking recipes and food images. *IEEE Transactions on Pattern Analysis and Machine Intelligence* 43(1):187–203.

Martin, C. K., H. Han, S. M. Coulon, H. R. Allen, C. M. Champagne, and S. D. Anton. 2009. A novel method to remotely measure food intake of free-living individuals in real time: The remote food photography method. *British Journal of Nutrition* 101(3):446–456.

Martin, S. L., M. I. Cardel, T. L. Carson, J. O. Hill, T. Stanley, S. Grinspoon, F. Steger, L. T. Blackman Carr, M. Ashby-Thompson, D. Stewart, J. Ard, and F. C. Stanford. 2023. Increasing diversity, equity, and inclusion in the fields of nutrition and obesity: A roadmap to equity in academia. *American Journal of Clinical Nutrition* 117(4):659–671.

McClung, H. L., H. A. Raynor, S. L. Volpe, J. T. Dwyer, and C. Papoutsakis. 2022. A primer for the evaluation and integration of dietary intake and physical activity digital measurement tools into nutrition and dietetics practice. *Journal of the Academy of Nutrition and Dietetics* 122(1):207–218.

McDonald, D., Y. Jiang, M. Balaban, K. Cantrell, Q. Zhu, A. Gonzalez, J. T. Morton, G. Nicolaou, D. H. Parks, S. M. Karst, M. Albertsen, P. Hugenholtz, T. DeSantis, S. J. Song, A. Bartko, A. S. Havulinna, P. Jousilahti, S. Cheng, M. Inouye, T. Niiranen, M. Jain, V. Salomaa, L. Lahti, S. Mirarab, and R. Knight. 2023. Greengenes2 unifies microbial data in a single reference tree. *Nature Biotechnology*. https://doi.org/10.1038/s41587-023-01845-1.

Mentzer, J. T., W. DeWitt, J. S. Keebler, S. Min, N. W. Nix, C. D. Smith, and Z. G. Zacharia. 2001. Defining supply chain management. *Journal of Business Logistics* 22(2):1–25.

Metcalf, H., D. Russell, and C. Hill. 2018. Broadening the science of broadening participation in STEM through critical mixed methodologies and intersectionality frameworks. *American Behavioral Scientist* 62:000276421876887.

Mitsuyama, Y., T. Matsumoto, H. Tatekawa, S. L. Walston, T. Kimura, A. Yamamoto, T. Watanabe, Y. Miki, and D. Ueda. 2023. Chest radiography as a biomarker of ageing: Artificial intelligence–based, multi-institutional model development and validation in Japan. *Lancet Healthy Longevity* 4(9):e478–e486.

Modanwal, G., J. R. Walker, S. Al-Kindi, S. Rajagopalan, and A. Madabhushi. 2020. Abstract 16796: Machine learning-based hepatic fat assessment in low-dose coronary artery calcium scans is correlated with human reader assessment. *Circulation* 142(Suppl_3):A16796.

Müller, M. J., and A. Bosy-Westphal. 2020. From a "metabolomics fashion" to a sound application of metabolomics in research on human nutrition. *European Journal of Clinical Nutrition* 74(12):1619–1629.

Nirschl, J. J., A. Janowczyk, E. G. Peyster, R. Frank, K. B. Margulies, M. D. Feldman, and A. Madabhushi. 2018. A deep-learning classifier identifies patients with clinical heart failure using whole-slide images of H&E tissue. *PloS One* 13(4):e0192726.

Noriega, M., J. Larco, C. Antonini, and C. Mejia. 2021. Market size and direct accessibility as mediators for explaining potato prices. Paper read at MIT SCALE Latin America Conference for Latin America & the Caribbean. https://scale.mit.edu/sites/scale.mit.edu/files/MIT-SCALE-Latin-America-Caribbean-2020-2021-Proceedings-Abstracts.pdf (accessed December 26, 2023).

Oakden-Rayner, L., J. Dunnmon, G. Carneiro, and C. Ré. 2020. Hidden stratification causes clinically meaningful failures in machine learning for medical imaging. *Proceedings of the ACM Conference on Health Inference and Learning* 2020:151–159.

Obermeyer, Z., B. Powers, C. Vogeli, and S. Mullainathan. 2019. Dissecting racial bias in an algorithm used to manage the health of populations. *Science* 366(6464):447–453.

OECD (Organisation for Economic Co-operation and Development). 2019. *The heavy burden of obesity: The economics of prevention*. Paris: OECD Publishing. https://doi.org/10.1787/67450d67-en (accessed January 9, 2024).

Our World in Data. 2023. *Change in cereal production, yield, land use and population, world*. https://ourworldindata.org/grapher/index-of-cereal-production-yield-and-land-use (accessed January 9, 2023).

Pallmann, P., A. W. Bedding, B. Choodari-Oskooei, M. Dimairo, L. Flight, L. V. Hampson, J. Holmes, A. P. Mander, L. Odondi, M. R. Sydes, S. S. Villar, J. M. S. Wason, C. J. Weir, G. M. Wheeler, C. Yap, and T. Jaki. 2018. Adaptive designs in clinical trials: Why use them, and how to run and report them. *BMC Medicine* 16(1):29.

Pardey, P. G., and J. M. Alston. 2021. Unpacking the agricultural black box: The rise and fall of American farm productivity growth. *The Journal of Economic History* 81(1):114-155.

Päßler, S., M. Wolff, and W. J. Fischer. 2012. Food intake monitoring: An acoustical approach to automated food intake activity detection and classification of consumed food. *Physiological Measurement* 33(6):1073–1093.

Perry, A. M., M. Steinbaum, and C. Romer. 2021. *Student loans, the racial wealth divide, and why we need full student debt cancellation*. Washington, DC: Brookings Institute.

Pyrros, A., J. M. Rodríguez-Fernández, S. M. Borstelmann, J. W. Gichoya, J. M. Horowitz, B. Fornelli, N. Siddiqui, Y. Velichko, O. Koyejo Sanmi, and W. Galanter. 2022. Detecting racial/ethnic health disparities using deep learning from frontal chest radiography. *Journal of the American College of Radiology* 19(1 Pt B):184–191.

Pyrros, A., S. M. Borstelmann, R. Mantravadi, Z. Zaiman, K. Thomas, B. Price, E. Greenstein, N. Siddiqui, M. Willis, I. Shulhan, J. Hines-Shah, J. M. Horowitz, P. Nikolaidis, M. P. Lungren, J. M. Rodríguez-Fernández, J. W. Gichoya, S. Koyejo, A. E. Flanders, N. Khandwala, A. Gupta, J. W. Garrett, J. P. Cohen, B. T. Layden, P. J. Pickhardt, and W. Galanter. 2023. Opportunistic detection of type 2 diabetes using deep learning from frontal chest radiographs. *Nature Communications* 14(1):4039.

Qiu, J., F. P.-W. Lo, X. Gu, M. L. Jobarteh, W. Jia, T. Baranowski, M. Steiner-Asiedu, A. K. Anderson, M. A. McCrory, and E. Sazonov. 2023. Egocentric image captioning for privacy-preserved passive dietary intake monitoring. *IEEE Transactions on Cybernetics*. https://doi.org/10.1109/TCYB.2023.3243999.

Quinn, R. A., A. V. Melnik, A. Vrbanac, T. Fu, K. A. Patras, M. P. Christy, Z. Bodai, P. Belda-Ferre, A. Tripathi, L. K. Chung, M. Downes, R. D. Welch, M. Quinn, G. Humphrey, M. Panitchpakdi, K. C. Weldon, A. Aksenov, R. da Silva, J. Avila-Pacheco, C. Clish, S. Bae, H. Mallick, E. A. Franzosa, J. Lloyd-Price, R. Bussell, T. Thron, A. T. Nelson, M. Wang, E. Leszczynski, F. Vargas, J. M. Gauglitz, M. J. Meehan, E. Gentry, T. D. Arthur, A. C. Komor, O. Poulsen, B. S. Boland, J. T. Chang, W. J. Sandborn, M. Lim, N. Garg, J. C. Lumeng, R. J. Xavier, B. I. Kazmierczak, R. Jain, M. Egan, K. E. Rhee, D. Ferguson, M. Raffatellu, H. Vlamakis, G. G. Haddad, D. Siegel, C. Huttenhower, S. K. Mazmanian, R. M. Evans, V. Nizet, R. Knight, and P. C. Dorrestein. 2020. Global chemical effects of the microbiome include new bile-acid conjugations. *Nature* 579(7797):123–129.

Raghu, V. K., J. Weiss, U. Hoffmann, H. J. W. L. Aerts, and M. T. Lu. 2021. Deep learning to estimate biological age from chest radiographs. *JACC: Cardiovascular Imaging* 14(11):2226–2236.

Reedy, J., A. F. Subar, S. M. George, and S. M. Krebs-Smith. 2018. Extending methods in dietary patterns research. *Nutrients* 10(5).

Ribeiro, M. T., S. Singh, and C. Guestrin. 2016. "Why should I trust you?" Explaining the predictions of any classifier. Paper read at Proceedings of the 22nd ACM SIGKDD International Conference on Knowledge Discovery and Data mining. https://dl.acm.org/doi/10.1145/2939672.2939778 (accessed December 21, 2023).

Ritchie, H., P. Rosado, and M. Roser. 2022. *Environmental impacts of food production*. https://ourworldindata.org/environmental-impacts-of-food (accessed December 1, 2023).

Rock, D., and H. Grant. 2016. Why diverse teams are smarter. *Harvard Business Review*. November 4. https://hbr.org/2016/11/why-diverse-teams-are-smarter (accessed February 22, 2024).

Rudin, C. 2019. Stop explaining black box machine learning models for high stakes decisions and use interpretable models instead. *Nature Machine Inteligence* 1(5):206–215.

Rushing, B. R., S. McRitchie, L. Arbeeva, A. E. Nelson, M. A. Azcarate-Peril, Y. Y. Li, Y. Qian, W. Pathmasiri, S. C. J. Sumner, and R. F. Loeser. 2022. Fecal metabolomics reveals products of dysregulated proteolysis and altered microbial metabolism in obesity-related osteoarthritis. *Osteoarthritis and Cartilage* 30(1):81–91.

Russell, B. J., S. D. Brown, N. Siguenza, I. Mai, A. R. Saran, A. Lingaraju, E. S. Maissy, A. C. Dantas Machado, A. F. M. Pinto, C. Sanchez, L. A. Rossitto, Y. Miyamoto, R. A. Richter, S. B. Ho, L. Eckmann, J. Hasty, D. J. Gonzalez, A. Saghatelian, R. Knight, and A. Zarrinpar. 2022. Intestinal transgene delivery with native E. coli chassis allows persistent physiological changes. *Cell* 185(17):3263–3277.

Sabry, F., T. Eltaras, W. Labda, K. Alzoubi, and Q. Malluhi. 2022. Machine learning for healthcare wearable devices: The big picture. *Journal of Healthcare Engineering* 2022:4653923.

Saleiro, P., B. Kuester, L. Hinkson, J. London, A. Stevens, A. Anisfeld, K. T. Rodolfa, and R. Ghani. 2018. Aequitas: A bias and fairness audit toolkit. *arXiv preprint arXiv:1811.05577*. https://arxiv.org/abs/1811.05577 (accessed January 9, 2024).

Sanches, L. M., and C. Mejía Argueta. 2019. *Rethinking fresh food supply chains*. White Paper. MIT Center for Transportation and Logistics.

Sazonov, E. S., and J. M. Fontana. 2012. A sensor system for automatic detection of food intake through non-invasive monitoring of chewing. *IEEE Sensors Journal* 12(5):1340–1348.

Schwedhelm, C., L. M. Lipsky, G. E. Shearrer, G. M. Betts, A. Liu, K. Iqbal, M. S. Faith, and T. R. Nansel. 2021. Using food network analysis to understand meal patterns in pregnant women with high and low diet quality. *International Journal of Behavioral Nutrition and Physical Activity* 18(1):101.

Seyyed-Kalantari, L., H. Zhang, M. B. McDermott, I. Y. Chen, and M. Ghassemi. 2021. Underdiagnosis bias of artificial intelligence algorithms applied to chest radiographs in under-served patient populations. *Nature Medicine* 27(12):2176–2182.

Shah, N., G. Srivastava, D. W. Savage, and V. Mago. 2019. Assessing Canadians health activity and nutritional habits through social media. *Frontiers in Public Health* 7:400.

Snoek, H. M., L. M. T. Eijssen, M. Geurts, C. Vors, K. A. Brown, M.-J. Bogaardt, R. A. M. Dhonukshe-Rutten, C. T. Evelo, L. K. Fezeu, P. M. Finglas, M. Laville, M. Ocké, G. Perozzi, K. Poppe, N. Slimani, I. Tetens, L. Timotijevic, K. Zimmermann, and P. van 't Veer. 2018. Advancing food, nutrition, and health research in Europe by connecting and building research infrastructures in a DISH-RI: Results of the Eurodish project. *Trends in Food Science & Technology* 73:58–66.

Sohn, J. H., Y. Chen, D. Lituiev, J. Yang, K. Ordovas, D. Hadley, T. H. Vu, B. L. Franc, and Y. Seo. 2022. Prediction of future healthcare expenses of patients from chest radiographs using deep learning: A pilot study. *Scientific Reports* 12(1):8344.

Sørensen, C. G., S. Fountas, E. Nash, L. Pesonen, D. Bochtis, S. M. Pedersen, B. Basso, and S. B. Blackmore. 2010. Conceptual model of a future farm management information system. *Computers and Electronics in Agriculture* 72(1):37–47.

Spencer, C. N., J. L. McQuade, V. Gopalakrishnan, J. A. McCulloch, M. Vetizou, A. P. Cogdill, M. A. W. Khan, X. Zhang, M. G. White, C. B. Peterson, M. C. Wong, G. Morad, T. Rodgers, J. H. Badger, B. A. Helmink, M. C. Andrews, R. R. Rodrigues, A. Morgun, Y. S. Kim, J. Roszik, K. L. Hoffman, J. Zheng, Y. Zhou, Y. B. Medik, L. M. Kahn, S. Johnson, C. W. Hudgens, K. Wani, P. O. Gaudreau, A. L. Harris, M. A. Jamal, E. N. Baruch, E. Perez-Guijarro, C. P. Day, G. Merlino, B. Pazdrak, B. S. Lochmann, R. A. Szczepaniak-Sloane, R. Arora, J. Anderson, C. M. Zobniw, E. Posada, E. Sirmans, J. Simon, L. E. Haydu, E. M. Burton, L. Wang, M. Dang, K. Clise-Dwyer, S. Schneider, T. Chapman, N. A. S. Anang, S. Duncan, J. Toker, J. C. Malke, I. C. Glitza, R. N. Amaria, H. A. Tawbi, A. Diab, M. K. Wong, S. P. Patel, S. E. Woodman, M. A. Davies, M. I. Ross, J. E. Gershenwald, J. E. Lee, P. Hwu, V. Jensen, Y. Samuels, R. Straussman, N. J. Ajami, K. C. Nelson, L. Nezi, J. F. Petrosino, P. A. Futreal, A. J. Lazar, J. Hu, R. R. Jenq, M. T. Tetzlaff, Y. Yan, W. S. Garrett,

C. Huttenhower, P. Sharma, S. S. Watowich, J. P. Allison, L. Cohen, G. Trinchieri, C. R. Daniel, and J. A. Wargo. 2021. Dietary fiber and probiotics influence the gut microbiome and melanoma immunotherapy response. *Science* 374(6575):1632–1640.

Sumner, S. C. J., S. McRitchie, and W. Pathmasiri. 2020. Chapter 10—Metabolomics for biomarker discovery and to derive genetic links to disease. In *Principles of nutrigenetics and nutrigenomics*, edited by R. D. E. Caterina, J. A. Martinez and M. Kohlmeier. Academic Press. Pp. 75–79.

Sun, M., L. E. Burke, Z. H. Mao, Y. Chen, H. C. Chen, Y. Bai, Y. Li, C. Li, and W. Jia. 2014. Ebutton: A wearable computer for health monitoring and personal assistance. *Proceedings of the 37th Annual Design Automation Conference* 2014:1–6.

Ten Hagen, K. G., C. Wolinetz, J. A. Clayton, and M. A. Bernard. 2022. Community voices: NIH working toward inclusive excellence by promoting and supporting women in science. *Nature Communications* 13(1):1682.

Topol, E. J. 2014. Individualized medicine from prewomb to tomb. *Cell* 157(1):241–253.

Verma, M., R. Hontecillas, N. Tubau-Juni, V. Abedi, and J. Bassaganya-Riera. 2018. Challenges in personalized nutrition and health. *Frontiers in Nutrition* 5.

Vrbanac, A., K. A. Patras, A. K. Jarmusch, R. H. Mills, S. R. Shing, R. A. Quinn, F. Vargas, D. J. Gonzalez, P. C. Dorrestein, R. Knight, and V. Nizet. 2020. Evaluating organism-wide changes in the metabolome and microbiome following a single dose of antibiotic. *mSystems* 5(5).

Wegge, J., F. Jungmann, S. Liebermann, M. Shemla, B. C. Ries, S. Diestel, and K. H. Schmidt. 2012. What makes age diverse teams effective? Results from a six-year research program. *Work* 41 (Suppl 1):5145–5151.

Williams, D., and G. Shipley. 2021. Enhancing artificial intelligence with indigenous wisdom. *Open Journal of Philosophy* 11:43–58.

Wu, E., K. Wu, R. Daneshjou, D. Ouyang, D. E. Ho, and J. Zou. 2021a. How medical AI devices are evaluated: Limitations and recommendations from an analysis of FDA approvals. *Nature Medicine* 27(4):582–584.

Wu, X., X. Fu, Y. Liu, E.-P. Lim, S. C. Hoi, and Q. Sun. 2021b. A large-scale benchmark for food image segmentation. Paper read at *Proceedings of the 29th ACM International Conference on Multimedia*. Chengdu, China.

Xu, J., L. Xiang, Q. Liu, H. Gilmore, J. Wu, J. Tang, and A. Madabhushi. 2016. Stacked sparse autoencoder (SSAE) for nuclei detection on breast cancer histopathology images. *IEEE Transactions on Medical Imaging* 35(1):119–130.

Yang, X., A. Doulah, M. Farooq, J. Parton, M. A. McCrory, J. A. Higgins, and E. Sazonov. 2019. Statistical models for meal-level estimation of mass and energy intake using features derived from video observation and a chewing sensor. *Scientific Reports* 9(1):45.

Yang, Y., T. Y. Tian, T. K. Woodruff, B. F. Jones, and B. Uzzi. 2022. Gender-diverse teams produce more novel and higher-impact scientific ideas. *Proceedings of the National Academy of Sciences of the United States of America* 119(36):e2200841119.

Yatsunenko, T., F. E. Rey, M. J. Manary, I. Trehan, M. G. Dominguez-Bello, M. Contreras, M. Magris, G. Hidalgo, R. N. Baldassano, A. P. Anokhin, A. C. Heath, B. Warner, J. Reeder, J. Kuczynski, J. G. Caporaso, C. A. Lozupone, C. Lauber, J. C. Clemente, D. Knights, R. Knight, and J. I. Gordon. 2012. Human gut microbiome viewed across age and geography. *Nature* 486(7402):222–227.

Yu, Z., A. De Vries, Y. Ampatzidis, and D. D. Sokol. 2021. Who owns and controls farming data. *AE564/AE564* 10(5):2021.

Zeevi, D., T. Korem, N. Zmora, D. Israeli, D. Rotshchild, A. Weinberger, O. Ben-Yacov, D. Lador, T. Avnit-Sagi, M. Lotan-Pompan, J. Suez, J. Mahdi, E. Matot, G. Malka, N. Kosower, M. Rein, G. Zilberman-Schapira, L. Dohnalová, M. Pevsner-Fischer, and E. Segal. 2015. Personalized nutrition by prediction of glycemic responses. *Cell* 163:1079–1094.

Zhang, X., H. Dou, T. Ju, J. Xu, and S. Zhang. 2016. Fusing heterogeneous features from stacked sparse autoencoder for histopathological image analysis. *IEEE Journal of Biomedical and Health Informatics* 20(5):1377–1383.

Zuffa, S., R. Schmid, A. Bauermeister, P. W. P. Gomes, A. M. Caraballo-Rodriguez, Y. El Abiead, A. T. Aron, E. C. Gentry, J. Zemlin, M. J. Meehan, N. E. Avalon, R. H. Cichewicz, E. Buzun, M. C. Terrazas, C.-Y. Hsu, R. Oles, A. V. Ayala, J. Zhao, H. Chu, M. C. M. Kuijpers, S. L. Jackrel, F. Tugizimana, L. P. Nephali, I. A. Dubery, N. E. Madala, E. A. Moreira, L. V. Costa-Lotufo, N. P. Lopes, P. Rezende-Teixeira, P. C. Jimenez, B. Rimal, A. D. Patterson, M. F. Traxler, R. de Cassia Pessotti, D. Alvarado-Villalobos, G. Tamayo-Castillo, P. Chaverri, E. Escudero-Leyva, L.-M. Quiros-Guerrero, A. J. Bory, J. Joubert, A. Rutz, J.-L. Wolfender, P.-M. Allard, A. Sichert, S. Pontrelli, B. S. Pullman, N. Bandeira, W. H. Gerwick, K. Gindro, J. Massana-Codina, B. C. Wagner, K. Forchhammer, D. Petras, N. Aiosa, N. Garg, M. Liebeke, P. Bourceau, K. B. Kang, H. Gadhavi, L. P. S. de Carvalho, M. S. dos Santos, A. I. Pérez-Lorente, C. Molina-Santiago, D. Romero, R. Franke, M. Brönstrup, A. V. P. de León, P. B. Pope, S. L. La Rosa, G. La Barbera, H. M. Roager, M. F. Laursen, F. Hammerle, B. Siewert, U. Peintner, C. Licona-Cassani, L. Rodriguez-Orduña, E. Rampler, F. Hildebrand, G. Koellensperger, H. Schoeny, K. Hohenwallner, L. Panzenboeck, R. Gregor, E. C. O'Neill, E. T. Roxborough, J. Odoi, N. J. Bale, S. Ding, J. S. S. Damsté, X. L. Guan, J. J. Cui, K.-S. Ju, D. B. Silva, F. M. R. Silva, G. F. da Silva, H. H. F. Koolen, C. Grundmann, J. A. Clement, H. Mohimani, K. Broders, K. L. McPhail, S. E. Ober-Singleton, C. M. Rath, D. McDonald, R. Knight, M. Wang, and P. C. Dorrestein. 2023. A taxonomically-informed mass spectrometry search tool for microbial metabolomics data. *bioRxiv* 2023.07.20.549584. https://doi.org/10.1101/2023.07.20.549584.

A

Workshop Agenda

THE ROLE OF ADVANCED COMPUTATION,
PREDICTIVE TECHNOLOGIES, AND BIG DATA ANALYTICS
RELATED TO FOOD AND NUTRITION RESEARCH: A WORKSHOP

AGENDA

October 10–11, 2023

National Academy of Sciences Building
2101 Constitution Avenue NW
Washington, DC 20418

Virtual Webcast

Workshop Goals:

- Explore opportunities and challenges related to the application of advanced computation, big data analytics, and high-performance computing to support advances in food systems and nutrition research.
- Discuss the appropriate use of evidence generated through advanced computation, big data analytics, and high-performance computing to inform food- and nutrition-related programs and policies.
- Consider ethical considerations associated with advanced computation, big data analytics, and high-performance computing and strategies to mitigate ethical concerns and avoid bias.

- Identify opportunities and challenges related to capacity building and training to support robust and ethical application of advanced computation, big data analytics, and high-performance computing in food and nutrition research.

DAY 1: TUESDAY, OCTOBER 10, 2023
Location: LECTURE ROOM

9:00 AM   **Welcome**
Rodolphe Barrangou, North Carolina State University; Planning Committee Cochair

9:05 AM   **Introductory Remarks**
Patrick Stover, Institute for Advancing Health through Agriculture at Texas A&M University
Cindy Davis, U.S. Department of Agriculture, Agricultural Research Service
Jennifer Tiller, Deputy Staff Director, U.S. House Committee on Agriculture
Sharon Kirkpatrick, University of Waterloo; Planning Committee Cochair

9:45 AM   **SESSION I: Setting the Stage**
Moderator: Rodolphe Barrangou

Speakers:
The Current State of Advanced Computation, Big Data Analytics, and High-Performance Computing
Anant Madabhushi, Emory University and Georgia Tech

Ethics, Privacy, Bias, and Trust in the Application of AI
Judy Gichoya, Emory University

10:45 AM   **BREAK**

11:00 AM   **SESSION I: Setting the Stage, CONTINUED**

AI in Nutrition and Food Sciences: Promises and Challenges
Benoît Lamarche, Université Laval

Moderated Discussion

12:00 PM	LUNCH BREAK
12:50 PM	**SESSION 2: Applications and Lessons Learned, Part 1** Moderator: Sharon Kirkpatrick Speakers: **Applications and Lessons Learned: Wearables** *Edward Sazonov, University of Alabama* **Applications and Lessons Learned: Microbiome** *Rob Knight, University of California, San Diego (virtual)* **Applications and Lessons Learned: Metabolomics** *Susan McRitchie, University of North Carolina at Chapel Hill*
2:25 PM	BREAK
2:40 PM	**SESSION 2: Applications and Lessons Learned, Part 1 CONTINUED** Discussant: *Holly Nicastro, NIH Office of Nutrition Research* Moderated Discussion
3:20 PM	**SESSION 3: Capacity Building** Moderator: Carmen Tekwe, Indiana University in Bloomington; Planning Committee Member Speakers: **NIH Supported Training Program in Artificial Intelligence and Precision Nutrition at Cornell: Plans and the Road Ahead** *Saurabh Mehta, Cornell University (virtual)* **Inclusive Teams for Food and Nutrition Research** *Angela Odoms-Young, Cornell University* Moderated Discussion
5:00 PM	ADJOURN DAY 1

DAY 2: WEDNESDAY, OCTOBER 11, 2023
Location: ROOM 125

9:00 AM   Key Themes from Day 1 and Issues That Warrant Further Discussion
Diana Thomas, U.S. Military Academy at West Point; Planning Committee Member

9:20 AM   SESSION 4: Applications and Lessons Learned, Part 2
Moderator: Rodolphe Barrangou

Speakers:
Applications of AI in Food and Nutrition Research
Benoît Lamarche, Université Laval

Designing Nutrition Studies for AI Data Analysis
Sai Das, Jean Mayer USDA Human Nutrition Research Center on Aging at Tufts University

Farmers Trust in AI
Aaron Smith, University of California, Davis

10:50 AM   BREAK

11:05 AM   SESSION 4: Applications and Lessons Learned, Part 2 CONTINUED

Application of AI: Supply Chains
Christopher Mejía, MIT Center for Transportation and Logistics (virtual)

Discussant: *Elenna Dugundji, MIT Center for Transportation and Logistics*
Discussant: *Becca Jablonski, Colorado State University;* Planning Committee Member

Moderated Discussion

12:25 PM   LUNCH BREAK

1:10 PM   SESSION 5: Potential Applications of AI to Large-Scale Food
           and Nutrition Initiatives
           Moderator: Diana Thomas

           Speakers:
           Bridge to AI, Nutrition for Precision Health
           *Chris Hartshorn, NIH National Center for Advancing
               Translational Sciences (virtual)*

           Considerations for Ethics and Diverse Populations
           Janie Hipp, Native Agriculture Financial Services (virtual)

           Moderated Discussion

2:15 PM   SESSION 6: Final Discussion and Synthesis
           Moderator: Sharon Kirkpatrick

           Panel Discussion
           *Rodolphe Barrangou (Planning Committee Member)
           Sai Das, Christopher Mejía (virtual), Angela Odoms-Young
               (Workshop Speakers)*

3:00 PM   WORKSHOP ADJOURNS

This event was planned by the following experts: Rodolphe Barrangou, North Carolina State University (Planning Committee Cochair); Sharon Kirkpatrick, University of Waterloo (Planning Committee Cochair); Becca Jablonski, Colorado State University; Anant Madabhushi, Emory University; Carmen Tekwe, Indiana University; and Diana Thomas, United States Military Academy at West Point.

The planning committee's role is limited to organizing the event. A proceeding based on the event will be prepared by an independent rapporteur.

B

Biographical Sketches of the Speakers and Moderators

Rodolphe Barrangou, Ph.D., is the T. R. Klaenhammer Distinguished Professor at North Carolina State University (NC State). Dr. Barrangou is focusing on characterizing CRISPR-Cas systems and their applications in bacteria, especially to study and develop probiotics, including for genotyping, phage resistance, screening, genome editing, and antimicrobials. He spent 9 years at Danisco and DuPont and has been at NC State since 2013. For his CRISPR work, he received several international awards, notably the Canada Gairdner International Award, and was elected to the National Academy of Sciences, National Academy of Engineering, and National Academy of Inventors. Dr. Barrangou earned a B.S. in biological sciences from Rene Descartes University, France, an M.S. in biological engineering from the University of Technology in Compiegne, France, an M.S. in food science from NC State, a Ph.D. in genomics from NC State, and an M.B.A. from the University of Wisconsin–Madison. He is also the former chair of the board of Caribou Biosciences, a cofounder of Intellia Therapeutics, Locus Biosciences, TreeCo, Ancilia Biosciences and CRISPR Biotechnologies, an advisor to Inari Ag, Invaio, Provaxus, Felix Biotech, the IGI, and editor in chief of *CRISPR Journal*.

Sai Krupa Das, Ph.D., is a senior scientist on the Energy Metabolism Team at the Jean Mayer USDA [U.S. Department of Agriculture] Human Nutrition Research Center on Aging and professor at the Friedman School of Nutrition Science and Policy, both at Tufts University. She has more than 20 years of experience in human nutrition research and in the field of energy metabolism. She has examined energy expenditure in adults with varying weight status and is an expert on doubly labeled water and other methodologies for measuring energy intake and expenditure and body composition. Dr. Das has conducted several clinical trials involving lifestyle interventions for attenuating age-related changes and targeting the obesity epidemic, including employees at worksites, hard-to-reach segments of the general population, military families, and people from around the world who face weight-related health challenges. She is widely published for her ongoing work on the landmark Comprehensive Assessment of Long-Term Effects of Reducing Intake of Energy trial, the first and largest randomized controlled trial of calorie restriction in humans. Her publications include *A Standard Calculation Methodology for Human Doubly Labeled Water Studies, Evaluation of PIQNIQ, a Novel Mobile Application for Capturing Dietary Intake,* and *Opportunities and Challenges of Technology Tools in Dietary and Activity Assessment: Bridging Stakeholder Viewpoints.* Dr. Das is executive director of the International Weight Control Registry, clinical center principal investigator (PI) and cochair of the Nutrition for Precision Health (NPH) Consortium, and a member of the Energy and Macronutrient Metabolism Research Interest Group of the American Society of Nutrition, Obesity Society, and Gerontological Society of America. Dr. Das holds a Ph.D. in human nutrition from the Friedman School of Nutrition Science and Policy.

Cindy D. Davis, Ph.D., serves as national program leader for the USDA-ARS in human nutrition program, where she helps direct the scientific program for six Human Nutrition Research Centers. Earlier, she was the director of Grants and Extramural Activities in the Office of Dietary Supplements (ODS), where she actively engaged and encouraged partnerships with other National Institutes of Health (NIH) institutes and centers to develop a portfolio that advances both nutritional and botanical dietary supplement research for optimizing public health. Dr. Davis is also actively involved in a number of government working groups focused on the microbiome, including as a cofounder and cochair of the Joint Agency Microbiome (NIH, Food and Drug Administration, National Institute of Standards and Technology, and USDA) working group. Before ODS, she was a program director in the Nutritional Sciences Research Group at the National Cancer Institute (NCI). She completed her postdoctoral training at the Laboratory of Experimental Carcinogenesis at NCI and joined the Grand Forks Human Nutrition Research Center, USDA, as a research nutritionist. In 2000, she received a Presidential Early Career Award for Scientists and Engineers and was named the USDA Early Career Scientist. She has published more than 135 peer-reviewed journal articles and 11 invited book chapters. She is a supplement editor for the *Journal of Nutrition*, assistant editor for *Nutrition Reviews*, and member of the editorial board for *Advances in Nutrition*.

Dr. Davis received her B.S. in nutritional sciences with honors from Cornell University in Ithaca, NY, and her Ph.D. in nutrition with a minor in human cancer biology from the University of Wisconsin–Madison.

Elenna Dugundji, Ph.D., is a research scientist at the Massachusetts Institute of Technology (MIT) Center for Transportation and Logistics. She shapes supply chain futures by bringing expertise in demand forecasting, machine learning (ML), and artificial intelligence (AI) to research in mainport logistics, involving network analytics, optimization of operational processes, tactical planning and strategic asset management. She received her Ph.D. in environmental sciences from the University of Amsterdam.

Judy Gichoya, M.D., is an associate professor at Emory University in interventional radiology and informatics. Her career focus is on validating ML models for health in real clinical settings, exploring explainability, fairness, and specifically how algorithms fail. She is heavily invested in training the next generation of data scientists through multiple high school programs. At Emory, she is the program director for radiology, sits on the AI Humanity Advisory Group, serves on the AI trainee editorial board, and teaches the medical students' ML elective.

Chris Hartshorn, Ph.D., is the chief of the Digital & Mobile Technologies Section and acting chief of the Clinical and Translational Science Awards Program Branch within the National Center for Advancing Translational Sciences Division of Clinical Innovation, where he manages and coordinates programmatic and research activities. Earlier, he served as a program director in the NCI Division of Cancer Treatment and Diagnosis. During his tenure at NIH, he has guided and managed multiple programs, including its Academic–Industrial Partnerships, NPH, and Bridge to Artificial Intelligence. Through these programs, he established the AI for Multimodal Data Modeling and Bioinformatics Center and several corollary efforts for the NCI Strategic Plan for AI/ML in Cancer. A principal focus has been creating initiatives to bring more care to more patients remotely via sophisticated multimodal analytical methods, AI, and novel biomedical technologies. Before NIH, he was a research staff member at the National Institute of Standards and Technology for projects focused on biomedical and national security applications and then collaborations with the U.S. Department of Defense, U.S. Department of Justice, NIH, Merck, and Pfizer.

Janie Simms Hipp, J.D., is the inaugural president and chief executive officer of Native Agriculture Financial Services, the first-ever Other Financing Institution within the Farm Credit System that will fund Native farmers and ranchers. She served as general counsel for the U.S. Department of

Agriculture, the first Native American in that role. She is the founder of the Indigenous Food and Agriculture Initiative at the University of Arkansas and the U.S. Department of Agriculture's Office of Tribal Relations in the Office of the Secretary and founding executive director of the Native American Agriculture Fund. She has also served on two delegations to the United Nations regarding women's and Indigenous issues. As an agriculture and food lawyer and policy expert, she focuses on the intersection of Indian law and agriculture and food law. She earned her J.D. from Oklahoma City University School of Law and an M.A. in agricultural law from the University of Arkansas School of Law.

Becca B. R. Jablonski, Ph.D., is the codirector of the Food Systems Institute at Colorado State University, an associate professor in the Department of Agricultural and Resource Economics, and a 2022–2023 US–UK Fulbright fellow. Her research investigates the roles of cities in leveraging food policies to achieve progress toward sustainable development (e.g., food and nutrition security, farm and ranch viability, regional economic development, and environmental sustainability), highlighting trade-offs of different policy approaches and interventions. She pays particular attention to the geographic dimensions of impacts; she undertakes disciplinary research and large-scale quantitative modeling projects and leads engaged community processes. She works at local, regional, national, and international scales. Among other honors, Dr. Jablonski won the 2020 Distinguished Extension/Outreach Program Award from the Applied Agricultural Economics Association and the U.S. Department of Agriculture's Abraham Lincoln Award (the U.S. Secretary of Agriculture's Honor Award). She holds a Ph.D. from Cornell University. She was a 2019 speaker/participant in the National Academies Food Forum Workshop on Innovations in the Food System: Shaping the Future of Food.

Sharon I. Kirkpatrick, Ph.D., is associate professor in the School of Public Health Sciences at the University of Waterloo. Dr. Kirkpatrick's research focuses on the intersections between nutrition, human and planetary health, equity, and policy, using a systems thinking lens. Much of her work is aimed at improving methodologies for measuring dietary patterns to foster robust evidence on how these influence human and planetary health and how to promote healthy and sustainable eating practices. She is a member of the Canadian Institutes of Health Research Institute of Nutrition, Metabolism, and Diabetes Institute Advisory Board and Health Canada Nutrition Science Advisory Committee. Dr. Kirkpatrick is a registered dietitian and holds a Ph.D. in nutritional sciences (2008) and M.H.Sc. in community nutrition (2002) from the University of Toronto, a B.A.Sc. in applied human nutrition (2000) from the University of Guelph, and a B.Kin. in kinesiology (1996) from McMaster University.

Rob Knight, Ph.D., is the founding director of the Center for Microbiome Innovation and professor of pediatrics, bioengineering, data science, and computer science and engineering at the University of California, San Diego (UCSD). His research has linked microbes to a range of health conditions, enhanced our understanding of microbes in many environments, and made high-throughput sequencing accessible to thousands of researchers worldwide. His lab has produced many of the software tools and laboratory techniques that enabled high-throughput microbiome science, including QIIME and UniFrac. He is cofounder of the Earth Microbiome Project, American Gut Project, and Biota, Inc., which uses DNA from microbes in the subsurface to guide oilfield decisions. He set up and runs the wastewater COVID-19 detection program and cofounded the COVID-19 testing lab at UCSD, which performs thousands of clinical tests per day and also sequences viral genomes out of wastewater and clinical samples. He is a fellow of the American Association for the Advancement of Science and American Academy of Microbiology and received the 2019 NIH Director's Pioneer Award and 2017 Massry Prize. Dr. Knight earned his B.S. in biochemistry from the University of Otago and his Ph.D. in evolutionary biology from Princeton University.

Benoît Lamarche, Ph.D., is a full professor at the School of Nutrition at Université Laval and scientific director and founder of the FRQS-funded NUTRISS. He has published more than 420 peer-reviewed papers on physiological, clinical, epidemiological, and public health issues related to food and health. He leads NutriQuébec, the largest population-based study on nutrition and health funded by the government of Quebec. He has contributed to training more than 70 MSc, Ph.D., and postdoc students. He has received numerous awards, including from the Quebec Society of Lipidology, Nutrition, and Metabolism (Prix des Fondateurs, 2013) and Canadian Nutrition Society (Centrum New Investigator Award, 2011, and Khursheed Jeejeebhoy Award, 2020). He has cowritten two books with the acclaimed chef Jean Soulard on the topics of nutrition, sports, and health. He is an Olympian (1984, 1988) in long track speed skating.

Anant Madabhushi, Ph.D., is the Robert W. Woodruff Professor of Biomedical Engineering and on the faculty in the Departments of Pathology, Biomedical Informatics, and Radiology and Imaging Sciences at Emory University. He is also a research health scientist at the Atlanta Veterans Administration Medical Center. Dr. Madabhushi has authored more than 475 peer-reviewed publications and has more than 100 patents issued or pending. He is a fellow of the American Institute of Medical and Biological Engineering, Institute for Electrical and Electronic Engineers (IEEE), and National Academy of Inventors. His work "Smart

Imaging Computers for Identifying Lung Cancer Patients Who Need Chemotherapy" was labeled by *Prevention Magazine* as one of the top 10 medical breakthroughs of 2018. In 2019, *Nature Magazine* hailed him as one of five scientists developing "offbeat and innovative approaches for cancer research." Dr. Madabhushi was named to the Pathologist's Power List in 2019, 2020, 2021, and 2022.

Susan McRitchie, M.A., M.S., is the lead biostatistician and program manager in the Metabolomics and Exposome Laboratory at the University of North Carolina–Chapel Hill (UNC–Chapel Hill) Nutrition Research Institute. She has more than 10 years of experience analyzing metabolomics and exposome data that support research in precision nutrition, precision health, and precision environmental health. Ms. McRitchie has experience analyzing data using a variety of methods, including quadratic growth curves, ordinal logistic regression, logistic regression, multiple linear regression, principal component analysis, orthogonal projection to latent structures discriminant analysis, structural equation modeling, and random forest. She is also the program coordinator for the Metabolomics and Clinical Assays Center in the NIH Common Fund NPH Consortium. Ms. McRitchie earned her M.A. in mathematics from the University of California, Los Angeles, and her M.S. in biostatistics from UNC–Chapel Hill.

Saurabh Mehta, M.B.B.S., Sc.D., is a physician with training and expertise in nutrition, infectious disease, epidemiology, and diagnostics. He is a faculty member in the Division of Nutritional Sciences, Cornell University and on its executive leadership team. Additionally, he also serves as the director of the Program in International Nutrition and the cofounding director of the new Center for NPH. He also coleads the NIH NPH Research Coordinating Center. The central theme of Dr. Mehta's research is the interplay between nutrition and disease, including facilitating field-friendly assessment for both, and elucidating how nutrition can be used as a modifiable risk factor for improving health and associated outcomes, often in the context of pregnancy and early childhood, through a combination of active surveillance programs, invention of point-of-care diagnostics, and randomized controlled trials primarily in resource-limited settings in India, Sub-Saharan Africa, and South America. His research program is supported by funding from NIH, the National Science Foundation, USDA, the U.S. Agency for International Development, the World Health Organization, and the Department of Defense, among others. Dr. Mehta is also the director of a new training program on AI and Precision Nutrition supported by NIH.

Christopher Mejía-Argueta, Ph.D., is a research scientist at the MIT Center for Transportation and Logistics. He is a supply chain specialist whose research focuses on improving the efficiency and flexibility of operations in multiple stakeholders, addressing changing purchasing patterns, and coupling these dynamic consumer profiles with the retail landscape. He founded and directed the MIT Food and Retail Operations Lab, a global, interdisciplinary research group that combats food malnutrition, reduces food waste, ensures food safety, empowers smallholder farming, and builds local, short food supply chains using data- and model-driven approaches. Dr. Mejía leads research networks and educational programs for Latin America and the Caribbean with top-ranked universities and research groups. He has more than 14 years of experience and has developed dozens of applied research projects for companies, nongovernmental organizations, multilateral funding sources, and governments in more than 12 countries on three continents.

Holly Nicastro, Ph.D., M.P.H., is a program director in the NIH Office of Nutrition Research, where she serves as coordinator for NPH, powered by the *All of Us* Research Program. In this role, she is responsible for overall management of the NPH consortium, progress toward the program's goals, and monitoring of interactions between the consortium and the external community. Dr. Nicastro holds a B.Sc. in nutritional sciences from Pennsylvania State University, a Ph.D. in molecular and biochemical nutrition from the University of California, Berkeley, and an M.P.H. from Johns Hopkins Bloomberg School of Public Health. She completed a postdoctoral fellowship with NCI's Cancer Prevention Fellowship Program, where she worked in the Nutritional Science Research Group.

Angela Odoms-Young, Ph.D. (she/her/hers), is the Nancy Schlegel Meinig Associate Professor of Maternal and Child Nutrition and director of the Food and Nutrition Education in Communities Program and New York State Expanded Food and Nutrition Education Program at Cornell University. Her research explores social and structural determinants of dietary behaviors and diet-related diseases in low-income and Black/Latinx populations and centers on identifying culturally appropriate programs and policies that promote health equity, food justice, and community resilience. Dr. Odoms-Young has more than 20 years of experience partnering with communities to improve nutrition and health and 200+ academic publications, book chapters, and presentations. She has served on numerous advisory committees and boards, including the National Academy of Sciences Food and Nutrition Board, Institute of Medicine committees to develop the nutrition standards for the National School Lunch Program/School Breakfast Program and revise the food packages provided in the Supplemental Program for Women, Infants, and Children, and Council on Black Health. Dr. Odoms-Young was also a member of the Board of the Greater Chicago Food Depository and is a member of the American Heart Association Chicago Metro Board, Grow Greater Englewood, and Blacks in Green. She is the inaugural Equity Visiting Scholar at Feeding America. Dr. Odoms-Young received her B.S. in foods and nutrition from the University of Illinois at Urbana-Champaign and M.S./Ph.D. in community nutrition from Cornell University. Additionally, she completed a Family Research Consortium Postdoctoral Fellowship examining family processes in diverse populations at Pennsylvania State University and University of Illinois at Urbana-Champaign and a Community Health Scholars Fellowship in community-based participatory research at the University of Michigan School of Public Health. Before joining Cornell, Dr. Odoms-Young served on the faculty at University of Illinois at Chicago in the Department of Kinesiology and Nutrition.

Edward Sazonov (IEEE M'02, SM'11) received a systems engineer diploma from Khabarovsk State University of Technology, Russia, in 1993 and a Ph.D. in computer engineering from West Virginia University, Morgantown, WV, in 2002. He is a James R. Cudworth Endowed Professor in the Department of Electrical and Computer Engineering at the University of Alabama, Tuscaloosa, AL, and the head of the Computer Laboratory of Ambient and Wearable Systems (http://claws.eng.ua.edu). His research interests span wearable devices, sensor-based behavioral informatics and methods of biomedical signal processing, ML, and AI. Devices developed in his laboratory include a wearable sensor for objective detection and characterization of food intake (Automatic Ingestion Monitor); a highly accurate physical activity and gait monitor integrated into a shoe insole (SmartStep, winner of Bluetooth Innovation WorldCup 2009); and a wearable sensor system for monitoring cigarette smoking (PACT). The research in his lab was recognized by several awards, including best paper awards and the president's research award at the University of Alabama. In 2020, Dr. Sazonov served as a Fulbright Distinguished Chair at the University of Newcastle, Australia. His research has been supported by NIH, National Science Foundation, National Academies, and state agencies, private industry, and foundations. Dr. Sazonov is a specialty chief editor for *Wearable Electronics* and *Frontiers in Electronics* and associate editor for several IEEE journals.

Aaron Smith, Ph.D., is the DeLoach Professor of Agricultural and Resource Economics at the University of California, Davis, where he has been since 2001. Originally from New Zealand, he earned his Ph.D. in economics from UCSD. His research addresses economic and policy challenges related to agriculture, energy, and the environment. He has more than 50 publications in refereed journals, including the *Review of Economics and Statistics*, *Journal of Econometrics*, *American Journal of Agricultural Economics*, and *Proceedings of the National Academy of Sciences*. His research has won the Quality of Communication, Quality of Research Discovery, and Outstanding *American Journal of Agricultural Economics* Article awards from the Agricultural and Applied Economics Association and Quality of Research Discovery Award from the European Association of Agricultural Economists. He is the cluster lead for socioeconomics and ethics in the AI Institute for the Food System.

Patrick J. Stover, Ph.D., is the director of the Institute for Advancing Health through Agriculture (IHA) at Texas A&M University, the world's first research institute to bring together precision nutrition, responsive agriculture, and behavioral research to reduce diet-related chronic disease in a way that considers environmental and economic effects. With support from USDA and Texas, the IHA includes an embedded USDA program. As an international leader in biochemistry, agriculture, and nutrition, Stover focuses on the biological mechanisms that underlie the relationships between food and human pathologies, such as birth defects, neuropathies, and cancer. He is an elected member of the National Academy of Sciences and a fellow of the American Association for the Advancement of Science. He is also former president of the American Society for Nutrition and served two terms on the National Academies Food and Nutrition Board. He received the Presidential Early Career Award for Scientists and Engineers from President Clinton, the highest honor bestowed by the U.S. government on outstanding scientists and engineers beginning their independent careers.

Carmen D. Tekwe, Ph.D., is an associate professor of biostatistics in the Department of Epidemiology and Biostatistics at Indiana University in Bloomington. She was a postdoctoral fellow and an assistant professor of biostatistics at Texas A&M University before joining Indiana University in 2019. Her research interests include developing statistical methodology to better assess big data, such as wearable-device-based measures, dietary intake surveys, and radiation risk assessments. She is the PI of a National Institute of Diabetes and Digestive and Kidney Diseases–funded R01 focused on statistical methods for measurement error correction in device-based measures of physical activity and self-reported dietary intake. She recently served as a consultant to the Committee on Dietary Reference Intakes Working Group at the National Academies. She is a scientific committee member of the National Council on Radiation Protection and Measurements Scientific Committee 1-28 and a member of the Scientific Leadership Council for the Institute for the Advancement of Food and Nutrition Sciences, an associate editor for *Statistics in Medicine*, and an ad hoc grant reviewer for NIH. She received both her B.A. and M.A. in statistics from the University of Florida and earned her Ph.D. in biostatistics from the University at Buffalo in 2011.

Diana M. Thomas, Ph.D., received her Ph.D. from the Georgia Institute of Technology in 1996. She completed a National Research Council–funded postdoctoral fellowship at the U.S. Military Academy and Army Research Laboratory. In 2000, she joined the faculty of Montclair State University, where she was a professor of mathematics and director of the Center for Quantitative Obesity Research. Dr. Thomas is a professor of mathematical sciences at the U.S. Military Academy at West Point. Dr. Thomas has been an active research mathematician for over 25 years, with a focus on nutrition and obesity related modeling. She is an associate editor for the world's top-ranked journal for original research in nutrition, *American Journal of Clinical Nutrition*, and coedits the series "Best (but oft-forgotten) practices," which consists of methodologic commentaries or statistical tutorials. Dr. Thomas is the PI of the Artificial Intelligence, Data Engineering, & Machine Learning Center for the NPH Consortium and cochair for the Steering Committee. She has held governance positions in the Obesity Society, American Society of Nutrition, and Mathematical Association of America.

Jennifer Tiller, M.P.A., M.B.A., serves as the deputy staff director for the House Committee on Agriculture under the leadership of Chair Glenn Thompson (R-PA). Ms. Tiller was both deputy staff director and senior professional staff for Chair K. Michael Conaway (R-TX). She has worked on a variety of legislative efforts affecting U.S. agriculture and domestic nutrition programs, including the 2018 Farm Bill, pandemic-related aid packages, and bills impacting federal spending and revenues. A Syracuse, New York, native, Ms. Tiller holds an M.P.A. from Marist College and M.B.A. from Syracuse University.